Holistic Approach

Holistic Network International

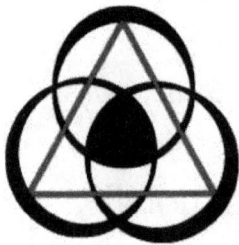

HOLISTIC
NETWORK
INTERNATIONAL

ISBN-13: 978-0692925317

HolisticNetworkInternational.com

Editor: Gina Carrillo

Cover: Rick Schettino

DEDICATION

This book is dedicated to holistic health professionals around the world who empower others to overcome physical and emotional challenges through mind, body, and spirit.

FOREWORD

For many, today's health-care is more accurately described as disease-care. I've heard of physicians who say they are trapped in the system. In order for their practice to survive, they must comply with insurance company requirements and leverage the perks of prescribing pharmaceuticals.

Physicians aren't the only ones who feel trapped in the system. For years, I dealt with chronic infection whose root cause was not a concern of the medical staff that I consulted. The system required me to make unnecessary appointments in order to continue receiving the "care" (prescriptions) they said would help me. They treated the symptoms, but did not offer me a solution for preventing the problem from recurring, leaving me feeling frustrated and helpless.

When I finally had enough, I took my health into my own hands and began reading as much as I could find on natural ways to deal with my health problems. I discovered natural remedies that did not threaten the health of my liver and kidneys, instead they nourished my body. I became so passionate about sharing this knowledge that I started teaching it to others. Eventually, I began connecting with practitioners who were doing the same. This book is a result of those connections.

Healing through mind, body, and spirit has been practiced for centuries. This book offers insight into a holistic approach to health and well-being. The pages that follow contain personal stories on approaches to wellness that consider a person as a whole, not isolated body parts and systems.

Imagine a heart-centered approach to health-care, where you have a relationship and trust with the person working with you to improve your well-being. Now more than ever, it is important to do your own research and empower yourself with knowledge so that you can make educated decisions about your health.

My hope is that this book, *Holistic Approach*, inspires and motivates readers to pursue a more holistic approach to wellness.

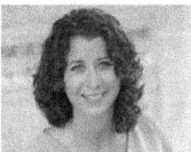

Sincerely,
Deserie Valloreo, Founder
Holistic Network International

CONTENTS

Foreword

1   Total Body Dental Health   1
Anthony J. Adams, DDS, PA

2   The Choice is Yours   7
Barry Foster, CRC, RCC, CPBA

3   Chronic Disease Resolution with Nutrition Therapy   13
Nwando Nwanna, Pharm.D

4   A Spiritual Journey to Becoming a Healer   19
Dr. Mark Tong

5   Journey to Well-being   25
Carla Clayton, CHC, Shaklee Distributor

6   Life Re-imagined   33
Clayton Sizemore, Certified Yoga Instructor, RYS-200, Travel
Professional

7   The Healing Road   39
Kimberly Dixson, Wholistic Health Coach, Yoga Instructor, Chinese
Herbalist

8   Farm Over Pharma   45
Vanessa Sardi, MS, CHE, CHC

9   Healing from Heartache and Learning to Love Myself   51
Anne Dort, Certified Clinical Herbalist, Holistic Health Coach

10   Wandering Paths   59
Lena Roberts, LMT, NMT

11   From a Mother's Heart: Unexpected Calling   65
Deborah R. Hutchinson, Functional Nutritionist, MS, BS, CHHC

12   Addiction Recovery - Transforming Darkness to Light   71
Jamey Kowalski, E-RYT200

13 Holistic Approach to Hormone Rejuvenation: Why the Cause and   77
    Solution for Hormone Imbalance is All Around Us
    Paige Clarke, CNHP, CA

14 The Quest for the Mind-Body Connection   83
    Gina Carrillo, Mind-Body Wellness Practitioner

15 Change Your Thoughts to Heal Your Life   91
    Terri Cabral, Certified Life & Business Coach, Spiritual Teacher

16 Survive and Thrive   97
    Saroep "Sara" Im, Award-winning Author, Speaker, Holistic Wellness
    Consultant

17 An Integrated Approach: The Road Less Traveled   103
    Lisa Seward, Licensed Massage Therapist MA10898, Certified
    BodyTalk™ Practitioner

18 Birth of My Son Led to 100% Organic Skincare Search   109
    Lucie Husarkova, Founder – Hug Your Skin 100% Organic Skincare

19 Holistic, Integrative Healing and Counseling   117
    Michael Whalen M.A., LMHC

CHAPTER 1

TOTAL BODY DENTAL HEALTH
by Anthony J. Adams, DDS, PA

Only ten years ago, I surveyed the new patients coming to my general dental practice located in Clearwater, Florida. Clearwater is part of the larger Tampa Bay community. Although I care for patients age 12 and up, the bulk of my patients are 40 and older. The socio-economic status of these patients crosses all strata. The majority live locally, that is within a 30-minute drive. However, I have more and more coming from distances as far as five hours away. Ten years ago, our intake forms surveying the patients understanding of the oral-systemic health connection showed one person in ten believing their oral health and their total body were related. Today, 49 out of 50 recognize there is a clear relationship between their oral health and their systemic health. There is a growing public knowledge and interest in this relationship. The Internet is changing the face of health. People are able to seek and find assorted and diverse paradigms in all aspects of health care and well-being. This may be challenging to established systems that currently have vested control, money, logistics, politics, and egos. This challenge is not without consequence. Regardless of benefits established belief systems may or may not have, they are slow to change because there is always resistance on so many levels.

Recently I saw reported an archeological dig, which uncovered a human tooth purported to be 13,000 years old. The tooth had been treated in much the same way as we would today. The decay had been removed using an implement, then the tooth had been filled with an herbal concoction covered with a clay filling. It is hard to understand why we have not advanced in our routine treatment protocols. It is more difficult to accept that current restorative dental protocols use toxic materials, which can have dire consequences. The questionable use of mercury amalgam as filling material has been debated for nearly 200 years. It is commonly accepted that mercury is extremely toxic. It is a neurotoxin. Consider how highly regulated and controlled the use of mercury is in every industry, except dentistry, where we commonly use it as filling material that is known to degrade. Nevertheless, we place it inches from the brain. Other than dentistry, every industry handles mercury as a bio-hazardous material, which is extremely toxic, easily absorbed by human tissue and most difficult to remove. I do not know which would be more binding, mercury to the bio-molecules of the human body or ignorance bound by traditions. I do not fault all dentists who have used mercury fillings. All dentists have been highly trained and indoctrinated in the belief they are doing a good thing. I was with the majority most of my career. I thought the material was wonderful to use, safe, and economical. I was wrong. I just did not know better. It was easy to use, but it was not wonderful for the patients I treated. It was not safe for them. Considering the cost to their systemic and oral health, I do not believe I could say it was economical. Today, without exception, I do not believe it should ever be used. I am equally passionate about how it is removed. My concerns are not only for the patient. The mercury vapor must be contained throughout the total office space to protect everyone. Our approved and proven protocol minimizes any biological risk. I believe a true and honest unbiased enquiry would make a substantial argument for these concerns. Politics may disagree. While we are on the subject of toxins, there are many materials with different degrees of toxicity that are currently being used in the mouth. The untoward effects may be minimal, undiagnosed, or misdiagnosed with some other symptoms. It is paramount each patient's full health history be reviewed, often with a fully qualified physician who will be working in concert with the dentist, but on the medical side of whole body health. I am not a physician licensed to provide medical care within our political delivery system. I work with a like-minded clinician who understands the duality of oral-systemic health. Holistic health considers the whole of a person. This concept of who we are is broad and deep. There are many levels and diverse modalities an individual holistic practitioner may have. Therefore, as individuals, we may agree or disagree between ourselves regarding the status of an individual patient and the best course of therapy for them. One thing you can always find in the holistic health arena is a seeker. One who seeks knowledge of "cause" over "symptom," I am committed to study and inquire each day. The paradox is, the more I learn, the less I know. When one is willing to let go of the very limiting dogma, the possibilities are exciting and addicting. I find it exciting to learn how important, life enhancing, and effective applied nutrition is to one's well-being. It is mind-boggling to consider the magnitude of other life forms that share one human body; even more amazing that we cannot exist without them. Much of our Newtonian-based therapies are designed with a "scorch and burn" mentality. "If this does not kill you, you may live" is ignorant. The knowledge we seek is how to find, create, then maintain homeostasis as individuals and as a collective. We share our bodies and our planet. Achieving balance...achieving homeostasis, should be the goal. It should not be not covering the symptoms by flipping switches that turn off the signals that indicate distress. We have by Divine design internal microbiomes that we are just beginning to understand. There are at back of your tongue, large papilla around which specific bacterium reside. When you rinse your mouth with a commonly-advertised mouth rinse that purports to kill 99.9% of all bacterium in your mouth, you kill all bacterium, including specific bacterium that produce nitric oxide, which is critically important in maintaining blood vessel flexibility. There are countless relationships in the mouth/body that seek balance, not "scorch and burn." When I initially see a patient with periodontal disease, or a lot of plaque, or osteoporosis, I know there is very likely a nutritional deficiency involving their calcium metabolism. With a calcium metabolism malfunction, they may very well have a problem with atherosclerosis. I see periodontal disease in over 50% of my new patients. I see undiagnosed thyroid disease in close to 20% of new patients. I know the presence of a mercury filling can cause imbalance in a person's thyroid. I work to identify materials in the patient's mouth that may hinder the physician's success at establishing homeostasis and thus health. Sixty percent of new adult patients I see are clinically dehydrated at their initial visit. This may be due to lack of water intake or consumption of some of the 400 commonly prescribed medicine patients take. Whatever the cause, dry mouth is an open door for oral disease. Oral disease is an open door for systemic disease. Optimal health is much more attainable than it seems. One must hydrate with quality water; alkaline is best. Eat healthy, exercise moderately, minimize stress, avoid toxic people and environments, detoxify your mouth and body, do not engage in habits, environments, people, or anything else that made you sick to begin with. And finally, seek help from clinicians who are willing to work out of the box, if necessary and with others who do the same. They should do this with your well-being; their goal and pleasure. We should never accept the status quo, if the status does not provide optimal results; in this case, optimal health. We should question, seek, and challenge that which does not provide an optimal result, even if it is tradition. At the same time, we must respect the pioneers and the truths left us. I provide below some of the pioneers and their books, which have influenced my path, both professionally and personally.

References

Huggins, H. (1993). *It's All In Your Head: The Link Between Amalgams and Illness*, (1999) *Uninformed Consent: The Hidden Dangers in Dental Car*

Rota, J. E. (2015). *Mirror of the Body: Your Mouth Reflects the Health of Your Whole Body*

Dental Surgeon

Malmstrom, C. (1996). *Chronic Fatigue*

Ziff, M. F. (2014). *Dentistry Without Mercury*

Galton, L. (1972). *The Laboratory of the Body*

Breiner, M. A. (2011). *Whole Body Dentistry: A Complete Guide to Understanding the Impact of Dentistry on the Total Health*

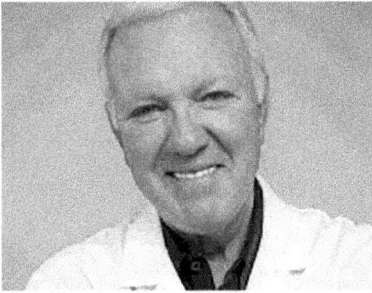

Dr. Adams attended the first dental college in the world, The Baltimore College of Dental Surgery, and graduated in 1976 with his Doctorate of Dental Surgery degree. He served in the Army Dental Corp. from 1976 to 1982, when he left to start his private practice. Dr. Adams has always been interested in the oral-systemic connection. His extensive studies convinced him one could not have optimal health or optimal oral health unless both were considered simultaneously. Therefore, he considers many health disciplines before he makes recommendations or treatment. Dr. Adams works with other health care providers in other disciplines to reach optimal health of each precious patient.

Dr. Adams' professional interest has always been the dynamic physiological relationship between the oral cavity and the rest of the body. He belongs to many organizations who promote knowledge in this connection, including:

ADA (American Dental Association)

IAOMT (International Academy of Oral Medicine and Toxicology)

ICIM (International College of Integrative Medicine)

AAEM (American Academy of Environmental Medicine)

IAMSD (International Association of Mercury Safe Dentists)

IABDM (International Academy of Biological Dentistry and Medicine)

HDA (The Holistic Dental Association)

DAMS (Dental Amalgam Mercury Solutions)

Price Pottenger Foundation

Holistic Network of Florida

Green People

Anthony J. Adams, DDS, PA
25877 US 19 North
Clearwater, FL. 33763
727-799-3123
www.healthybodydental.com

CHAPTER 2

THE CHOICE IS YOURS
by Barry Foster, CRC, RCC, CPBA

An excerpt from my book, *Overcoming Your Funk*, published in 2012:

The Choice is Yours ... *not just this choice, but every choice.*

Always remember this: every choice you make is in your control, not anyone else's.

> You can choose to stay where you are or you can choose to change.

> You can choose to believe in yourself again or you can choose to stay the victim.

> You can choose to change your attitude – or not.

Many of us have the mistaken attitude that we're forced into many of the choices we make, for example: *I have no choice. I must have this job because I need healthcare. My family gives me no choice but to...* The thinking is often something along these lines: *I have to endure what I'm enduring because of outside factors over which I have no control, and the choice to anything different is out of my hands.*

Most often, this is a myth. There are countless situations in which we feel we don't have a choice when in fact, we do. Let's say you have a 10:00 a.m. flight out of an airport that's 45 minutes away from your home. You make the choice to leave home one hour and forty-five minutes before flight time. On your way to the airport, you encounter stalled traffic, the result of an accident. Because of the delays, you arrive at the airport only 40 minutes before your flight time, so you choose to park in the parking garage, which costs twice as much as long-term parking. It was your choice not to consider possible delays on the way to the airport. You could have chosen to leave two hours and 15 minutes before flight time. As a result of your first choice, you made the second choice to park in the parking garage (twice as expensive), as opposed to missing your flight.

We may encounter outside influences. In the above scenario, we may not have been able to avoid the accident. We could not have prevented the traffic jam. We did, however, have a choice as to what time we left for the airport. We also have control over and choices as to how we react to any given set of circumstances.

Here's another example: think about how many times you've said something like, "Peter made me mad." Peter didn't make you mad. It was your choice to become mad about what Peter said or did. We have control over our emotions.

We have choice around what we're passionate about. We have the choice to discover our life purpose – or not. We chose how we act. We have the choice to reignite our spirit. We even have the choice to just lie on the sofa all day and do nothing. We have the choice to hunker down or get into action.

You might be thinking, *what about someone who gets sick with cancer? Was it a choice to get sick?* No one chooses to have cancer. However, there are choices we make in our lives that may contribute to ill health and ultimately cancer: smoking, eating junk food, being consistently overweight, not controlling stress. Some individuals choose to work in an environment in which they're exposed to carcinogens. Making poor choices when it comes to wellness may contribute to illness. Then of course there are those cases in which we hear of a seemingly perfectly healthy individual – who takes the best of care of herself – getting ill. In some cases, we may not have been able to prevent the cancer, but we have choices as to how we react to the tragedy of having cancer.

I recently saw a story on television of a 27-year-old female attorney with two small children. The attorney had a stroke and her doctors told her she'd never walk again. She made a choice: she chose not to believe those doctors and she was determined to walk again. She made a commitment to herself that she would learn to walk again, she would take care of her kids, and she would not be a burden to herself and others for the rest of her life. Two years later, she was walking, defying what her doctors had said.

We hear and read about medical miracles such as this all the time. You may even know someone who beat the odds. It all starts with making a choice. These people chose to *fight* back as opposed to *lay* back. Look around you and I promise you'll see examples of choices being made all the time. When you employ your choice to become bigger, better, faster, more productive, more energetic, more skilled at your job, more friendly, outgoing, and more receptive, those choices will drive you just as hard and just as far as the choice you can make to do nothing.

My story:

> On July 14, 2009 (more than 8 years ago), I made a choice to do whatever was necessary to take charge of my life. I chose to come up from being down in the dumps and to reignite my spirit. I chose to figure out how. I chose to reach out, take advice, and accept input and feedback from others. I had to make choices as to *what* I was going to change and *how* I was going to change.

> I had to make the decision that I was willing to do the hard stuff first. I chose to make a commitment to myself in writing. I chose to examine my lifestyle and keep what had been working and get rid of what was not working. These weren't easy choices because I wasn't at 100%. It takes patience, persistence, and practical application to climb out of the black hole.

> While I was making these changes and tough choices, I had to learn how to be happy and satisfied with where I was and where I was headed. I made the choice – and

the commitment – that I was not going back into a funk again. I made the choice that the quality of my future was right around the corner and I would keep my eyes on the horizon because that's where I was headed: forward, not backward.

Those are just some of the choices I had to make … and you will have to make them too.

I can report over the past eight years since making those choices, commitments, and changes, I'm living my best life ever. I'm healthier, happier, more fulfilled, more joyful, and my spirit has been reignited … and then some!

I hope you believe me now. The fact is, we *do* have choices – even when we don't think we do. This understanding is a key element to climbing out of the black hole. We must "own" those choices, hold ourselves responsible for our choices, and take accountability for them. When you've made a decision about something, be aware that you have made a choice – good, bad, or indifferent – accept your choice and embrace your choice.

When we finally come to understand that we have choices, we become more in control of our today and our tomorrow. Then we can change our inner conversation. We can change our mindset. We can choose to rise up instead of lay back.

So now you have a choice to make: do you want to take on the next step in climbing out of the black hole?

> "It's up to you to make choices that work best for you.
> It really is all within your point of view. Regret is a
> matter perspective. If you like who you are NOW, it
> follows that you can embrace, without regret, all the
> choices that led you here."

> *- Mary Anne Radmacher*

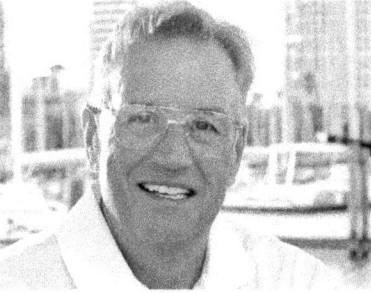

Barry Foster is a certified coach, workshop leader, career facilitator, author, speaker, and past radio personality with over 50 years of business experience. Trust, integrity, results, energy, leadership, excellence, support, and success are but a few of the values used to describe Barry. He is driven and passionate about helping everyone discover and overcome the barriers blocking them from achieving and enjoying both personal and professional success. His mission is to make a profound, positive, and significant difference in people's lives, every day. An avid cyclist, Barry lives in St. Petersburg, Florida with his wife, Penny.

Barry Foster, CRC, RCC, CPBA
bfoster@gmail.com
www.everyoneneedsacoach.com

CHAPTER 3

CHRONIC DISEASE RESOLUTION WITH NUTRITION THERAPY
by Nwando Nwanna, Pharm.D

My Personal Health Journey

I became a pharmacist because I was fascinated with how drugs could be used to heal diseases. I have been a practicing pharmacist for almost 20 years now, both as a clinical pharmacist in the hospital and a community pharmacist in a retail setting. In the course of my transition from hospital to community pharmacy setting, I realized that most of the drugs used to treat chronic diseases did not address the underlying cause of the disease. The drugs are used to suppress symptoms and prevent complications but did not offer a cure. I have also had some health issues that have not been resolved by drugs or conventional medicine, which led me to begin to search for alternative therapies.

I have had bowel problems for more than 10 years, as well as joint problems. I had tried all sorts of remedies without any cure. I would use anti-inflammatory drugs for my joint pain, but it bothered my stomach so I could only use it sparingly. I tried chiropractors, including advanced orthogonal chiropractors. I found relief for my lower back pain but it never lasted for more than three weeks. In fact, most of the time I would have to go weekly to the chiropractor to get adjusted. Early in 2015, I started experiencing extreme fatigue. It did not matter whether I slept or not, I woke up unable to get out of bed and when I forced myself up it was a drag to get through the day. I started some nutrition program with supplements that would help sometimes but never really resolved the issues. I knew that I was going through some pathology in my organ systems that no one had been able to identify.

One day, someone told me about Nutrition Response Testing. I decided to give it a try and was amazed at how the practitioner was able to identify the areas of my body that were not functioning well. My thyroid gland was identified as the priority, even though I had bowel, adrenal, and joint problems. It made sense to me because several months back, I had actually asked my doctor to test me for thyroid but the test came back normal. I had read so many articles that suggested that the standard test for thyroid function is not sensitive enough to identify thyroid dysfunction that was causing significant symptoms in people, especially women. I was also told I was sensitive to most grains and sugar. Again, I had already suspected these problems and had taken steps to structure my diet accordingly, but despite my healthy diet, I could not solve any of these problems that had plagued me.

I was put on a program that eliminated most grains and sugar. I was recommended whole food supplements that supported my thyroid and enzymes that not only helped with digestion, but helped me break down products that were in my system from previous diets that I could not break down. After a week on this program, I felt like a normal human being with normal energy. My bowel problems did not resolve that quickly but I was convinced right away that this was a program that produced results and I wanted to be part of it. I began to attend classes and training workshops to help me understand more about this system and ultimately to become a practitioner myself to help others.

I have been on the program since April 2015 and most of my health issues are now being resolved. I no longer have back pain, I am no longer fatigued for no reason, and my bowels are functioning once again. I no longer have to take NSAIDS or glucosamine chondroitin for joint pain. I still have problems with my knees if I run but I am confident that with time, that will also be resolved. It does take time for the body to rebuild itself and I will continue on the program to resolve all my health issues and to maintain my health.

Dietary Lifestyle for Health and Wellness

The majority of chronic diseases could be prevented through simple lifestyle changes. Some reports estimate that eliminating three risk factors: poor diet, inactivity, and smoking would prevent 80% of heart disease, 80% of type 2 diabetes, and 40% of cancer.

"The body has the potential to fully repair itself when given the right nutrients." This is a quote I believe is the guiding principle of natural healing. Our cell and tissues and organs are made up of combinations of molecules that are components of our food. So to repair any tissues we need "genuine replacement parts." Secondly, the chemical and electrical processes that occur in our body require binding of specific molecules to specific receptors to produce specific actions. It is not random. If we ingest substances that our body does not have binding receptors to match, or does not recognize, they will not produce any desired effect. Sometimes semi-synthetic compounds that resemble the natural molecule will bind partially to the receptors and produce only a partial effect and may even prevent the binding of the natural molecule for full effect. Thirdly, the detoxification processes in our body also requires binding of metabolic waste to specific receptors in the liver and other organs of elimination. Molecules that are not from nature will not be recognized and will not bind to those receptors. Therefore, detoxification through the normal process is impeded.

What Are the Nutrients Your Body Needs to Repair Itself?

Human beings by design are omnivores. This means we are capable of ingesting and digesting both plant and animal products. Macronutrients such as proteins, carbohydrates, and fats found in both plant and animal sources can be utilized by the human body.

We also need micronutrients, such vitamins minerals, and phytonutrients, which can be obtained from fruits and vegetables. Fermented foods are also important for probiotics needed for digestion.

Nutritional Therapies for Chronic Disease

When there is organ dysfunction, it is important to identify the root cause of the problem in order to eliminate it and give nutritional support for the organ.

Nutrition Response Testing is a non-invasive system of analyzing the body to determine the underlying cause of illness or non-optimal health. It uses a simple muscle test and neurological reflexes to assess how the autonomic nervous system is regulating the body's function for each organ.

Our program first identifies organs that are not functioning optimally using applied muscle testing, then identifies the root cause of the problem. The stressors or offending agents are removed by lifestyle changes, as well as with appropriate nutritional supplements. Whole food supplements are then used to support the organ to heal itself.

The cause of most health problems are:

- Food sensitivities or nutritional deficiencies
- Chemical and metal toxicities
- Immune challenges
- Other stressors

It is a simple process of removing the cause of the problem, the barriers to healing, and providing nutritional support for the organ. Everyone is different. So, it is important to use a process, such as muscle testing to identify and recommend specific nutritional program and supplements each individual needs for resolving the problem.

All Supplements Are Not Created Equal

It is also important to make the distinction between whole food nutritional supplements and synthetic supplements and processed foods.

Whole food nutritional supplements are derived from whole foods grown organically and minimally processed to preserve their vital enzymes and vitamins. Essential nutrients, such as vitamins, minerals, and phytonutrients exist as a chemical complex in nature. Some supplement manufacturers extract the active ingredient for use in their supplements. Some will use the active ingredient as a template to synthesize the vitamin. Many of these synthetic vitamins lack the transporters and co-factors associated with the naturally-occurring vitamins and so may not be utilized by the body as efficiently as natural vitamins. Synthetic vitamins may not contain the trace minerals required for processing of the vitamin and may use the body's reserve of minerals, leading sometimes to mineral deficiencies. They may be excreted if not utilized and the fat-soluble vitamins may accumulate in the body to dangerous levels.

I am happy to be able to offer clients a non-invasive, effective, natural healing method. One of my clients wrote: "My thyroid has been hypoactive for approximately 21 years and I have been taking an ever-changing dose of Synthroid daily. ......Fortunately for me I came across an AD for Wize Nutrition Therapy and Nutrition Response Testing. LIFE CHANGING!!!! Three months after a weekly customized Standard Process regimen, I was off all products including Synthroid and Thytrophin for my thyroid. My hair does not fall out like it did, not as dry or grey like it was. I do not experience the underactive thyroid 'brain fog' anymore. My vision improved... I have lost the 18 pounds that I had gained following surgery eight years ago!!! Thank you Nwando!!!"

This is the reason I am making the transition from a purely pharmacy practice to a pharmacy and nutrition based practice. I do understand that people need drugs for acute health conditions. Also, people with chronic diseases are not always able or willing to make the lifestyle changes and commitment required for natural healing with nutrition. I am proud to be a pharmacist that knows that drugs are not always the answer, and I am able to offer holistic viable options for healing.

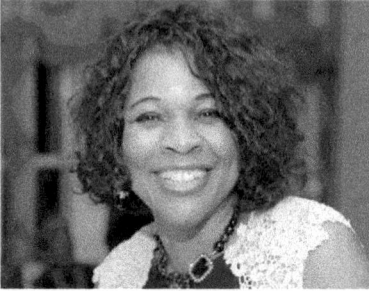

Dr. Nwanna graduated from the University of Florida, Gainesville in 1998 with a Doctor of Pharmacy degree. She worked as a clinical pharmacist in various hospitals in the Tampa Bay area for 10 years before starting her own community retail pharmacy. When she had health problems unresolved by medical therapy, she began to research alternative therapies that ultimately led her to train as a Nutrition Response Testing practitioner and establish a nutritional therapy practice in Florida.

Nwando Nwanna, Pharm.D
Wize Nutrition Therapy
34876 US HWY 19 N.
Palm Harbor, FL 34684
727-216-3972
wizenutritiontherapy@gmail.com
www.wizenutritiontherapy.com

CHAPTER 4

A SPIRITUAL JOURNEY TO BECOMING A HEALER
by Dr. Mark Tong

As a real estate broker in a family business, I found myself one morning in our conference room waiting to meet with one of my associates. As I sat there overlooking the garden in the atrium, just enjoying the moment, she walked in and I noticed she wasn't carrying any folders or files. She sat at the table across from me and said, "I am here to teach you the fundamentals for spiritual healing." Let's just say it was a little startling. The hair on the back of my neck stood up and goosebumps ran throughout my body. From that moment forward, she became my spiritual teacher. For nearly a year, I studied with her - a master teacher with a background in Christian healing.

It seemed the healing work I had been doing prior to this encounter was put on hold and I was being fine-tuned and taken to a new level. Then one day, I was referred to a wealthy individual who had been told he had cancer. This was the very first patient the teacher and I worked on together. Prior to meeting him, we both worked on him remotely. When I finally met the patient at his office, he was working on getting everything in order, as instructed by the doctors. As he spoke about his condition, I talked about his healing and that I saw him already healed. Having to overcome what the medical community had told him, I suggested he get a second opinion from the Mayo Clinic in Jacksonville Florida. Since he already had the highest respect for the clinic, whatever they said, he would know to be the truth. So, he packed his bags, medical reports, and x-rays and headed off to Jacksonville to hear these words: "no cancer found." That was over 25 years ago and the patient is still alive today, active and healthy.

So my life continued as a real estate broker and spiritual healer.

One evening as I was leaving the office, I received a phone call from someone who wanted to see one of our rental homes. With only a few minutes of daylight left, I scheduled to meet them promptly at the property. As I was racing across to my car, I took a shortcut through a planter bed in the parking lot. As I did, my foot hit the top of a tree root, landing me abruptly on my left shoulder. As I laid in the planter realizing what happened, I felt like I could barely move. After getting centered and pulling myself together, I was able to get up and get behind the wheel of my vehicle. In pain and partially paralyzed, I drove to the appointment. Despite the pain, I could still move so the showing of the property went well. The moment I got home, I went straight into meditation and within a few moments, all the pain was gone and I felt healed. However, the next morning when I woke, I could not move my entire upper body without being in pain. My business partner and I had a scheduled meeting that day to preview a piece of property we were looking to invest in. Knowing I could not drive, I called my partner and asked if he would drive me to the appointment. When he picked me up, he asked, "What happened?" I proceeded to give him a brief description of the event. Upon arrival to the building, we were greeted by my partner's wife, who was a former surgical nurse. My partner told her what had happened and she replied with a series of questions for me to determine the physicality of the issue. Because of my responses, she determined that I did something to my shoulder and it would require surgery and months of recovery. She then handed me a hand-written card where she had written the name and phone number of a doctor who specialized in these types of cases. After previewing the property, my partner and I returned to my office, at which time he stated, "You're not going to call anyone, are you?" Shaking my head "no" as I exited the vehicle, I worked my way back to my private office.

Shutting the door behind me, I sat at my desk, got centered and phoned a colleague of mine who does healing work similar to mine. Luckily, he answered the phone on the second ring. I briefly explained to him what had occurred and after a long pause he had this response: "Who else was with you when you fell?" I replied that I was alone and he quickly responded, "I am never alone" and "being one with God, only good can ever occur." The entire phone call was less than a few minutes and he agreed to work with me on the situation. The moment I hung up the phone, I went into a very calm and peaceful feeling and sat there for a few moments in a blissful state. My phone rang and without thinking, I picked it up with my left hand (the side that was injured) and answered it. As I was talking on the phone, I suddenly realized all the pain had dissipated and I had 100% movement on my entire left side. The healing was instantaneous. Later that weekend, I helped my brother move into a two-story apartment that did not have an elevator. Not only was the healing instant, but it was permanent.

In June 2007, something I had always anticipated would happen, finally occurred. The real estate market was at a record high with nothing supporting it. Like with every boom, comes a bust and this was it. The top of the real estate spiral had collapsed and everyone in the industry was being affected. Our office went from 44 agents to just four agents, almost overnight. I embraced the situation with the knowing that "it is all good." It was a cleansing and because of it, I could do what I came here to do - assist others in healing.

Our real estate office was merged with another office. This allowed me to exit the real estate brokerage industry and focus on the healing work. I worked non-stop making hospital visits, house calls, and office appointments. One day, I received a phone call from a former patient. She asked me if I was still doing healing work. As I replied "yes," she asked if she could begin to refer patients to me. Upon my favorable reply, I started to see those patients as well. What I did not realize at the time - they were referring me Stage IV cancer patients. After the first week of seeing these patients, I received another phone call from a former patient who asked if I would be willing to come to the clinic she worked at and meet the medical director. The meeting was brief, but we both realized we had parallel paths. At the conclusion of the meeting I asked, "Is there anything I can do for you?" The director led me to the back of the clinic and introduced me to a young female diagnosed with stage IV cancer. Immediately, I began working with her. At the end of the session, the medical director offered me the opportunity to "come and go as I wish and to do whatever I needed to do to assist the patients."

For nearly three years, I worked at this alternative cancer clinic as a spiritual counselor and healer. The clinic was more mainstream than those I had worked with in the past. Unlike what I had done in the past, here patients had different spiritual and religious backgrounds. Using the same approach I had learned from my spiritual teacher, I developed a system that takes an inventory of the patient's beliefs. By using it, along with kinesiology (muscle testing), I am able to identify the emotional events that led to the manifestation of the cancer. Remember, disease comes from not being "at ease." So, using the patient's own beliefs, I was able to bring them to peace, and it is in this peace that the body can begin to heal. While at the clinic, I published my findings and processes in my book, *Prevent Cancer.*

As I was working at the clinic, an individual my business partner and I had sold a property to prior to the real estate collapse defaulted on the mortgage and we were the underlying mortgage holders for the property. The property was the Crystal Bay Hotel in St. Petersburg, Florida. It is a 60-room historic hotel. When the former owner purchased the property, he gutted it in an attempt to convert it to a high-end boutique hotel. However, he got halfway through the renovations and ran out of money. When we received title to the property, my business partner was not in a position and did not want to move forward with renovating this property. This left us - with the property - at a standstill. Financially paralyzed, my partner suggested we split up our jointly-held properties. He would take the properties we held in New York and I would receive the properties in Florida, including the Crystal Bay Hotel. This was a quick and equitable solution we both agreed upon.

The moment I received the title to the to the hotel, I knew I would have to leave the clinic to free up the necessary time to reconstruct the hotel. One of the hardest days of my life was my last day at the clinic. Facing a major reconstruction and all the challenges that go with it, early one morning in meditation, I decided to make God my partner. With God as my partner, I knew I could not fail and everything I needed would be provided, and it was. Knowing I did not have the adequate funds to complete the project, I pressed on with the reconstruction. As I continued, everything I needed appeared: the workers, the materials, and even the funds. My mantra for the project was, "This is God's Hotel. Show me what to do next." If I ever felt challenged in a situation, I would just tell everyone involved that "they would have to deal with my partner."

In November of 2015, after two and a half years of construction, the hotel opened as a "Healing Hotel." At first, I thought we would be catering to cancer patients, like at the clinic, but the guests who were showing up were those who experienced emotional pain and trauma that had not yet manifested into any disease. Our focus quickly shifted to that of wellness by assisting others with physical and emotional healing, along with spiritual growth.

Throughout my healing work, I found with each and every patient, client and guest that I would refer to their situation as a "life lesson." One day in working with one of my students, when I used the term "life lesson," she asked me what the life lessons were. Not having a specific answer for her, I did something any spiritual teacher would do, I went to Google. To my surprise, Google, Wikipedia, and Amazon had no references to the real-life lessons. These lessons are the ones each and every person has to experience, and continue to experience, until "all levels of awareness become that of consciousness" and you reach a blissful, peaceful, and loving state of consciousness.

That night in meditation, I asked my partner, God, "What are the life lessons?" In a meditative state with a pen and paper in hand, I was given the "7 Life Lessons." When I compared the 7 Life Lessons to Dr. Bradley Nelson's, Emotion Code (a published chart that displays all of the negative, human emotions) and compared it to the Emotional Inventory Worksheet I developed at the clinic (it lists all of the emotional events that could be encountered), they matched. Even later on when I compared the 7 Life Lessons to the seven chakras, they matched.

Using kinesiology (muscle testing), I can quickly identify which lessons each person is still working on and tie the lessons to their own experiences or relationships, accelerating their spiritual growth, awareness, and healing. Not only did I utilize this process with my patients, clients, and guests, but I also put together a weekend retreat at the Crystal Bay Hotel in order to reach out and assist others on a larger scale. The retreat proved to be life changing for all who participated. So naturally, I began looking for another avenue to further assist people on an even grander scale. Thus, I have published the 7 Life Lessons online. For additional information, these lessons can be found at www.7LifeLessons.com.

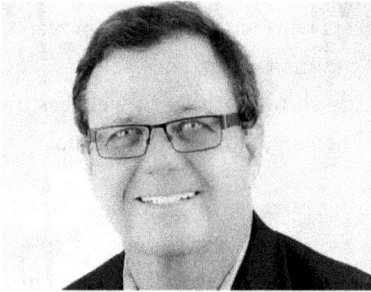

Spiritual healer/teacher of God, Dr. Mark Tong has had the opportunity to work with Stage IV cancer patients, where he developed a process to identify the underlying emotional events and trauma that manifested into the disease. Once this was brought to the patient's awareness, they then could begin to heal. He later identified these events as "life lessons" and discovered the "7 Life Lessons." These are the lessons that everyone must spiritually evolve through to obtain healing, inner peace, and spiritual enlightenment.

Dr. Tong assists individuals in physical and emotional healing, along with those seeking spiritual growth at the Crystal Bay Hotel in Saint Petersburg, Florida and online at 7LifeLessons.com.

CHAPTER 5

JOURNEY TO WELL-BEING
by Carla Clayton, CHC, Shaklee distributor

I suffered with allergies and chronic sinus infections for my whole life. My constant nasal drip was a problem for me since childhood. I went to many doctors, but I was a mystery diagnosis to all of them. They struggled to treat my allergies with pills and steroid sprays that never worked. One doctor told me to expect to be on antibiotics eight to nine months out of the year! By the time I was 26, I was just another stressed out school teacher who napped every day after work.

I had resigned myself to this life. I was a stressed, depressed mess. There was something missing from my life. Then a friend reached out to me and asked how I was doing. I agreed to meet up with her, hoping for some relief from my misery. I told her about my lifelong unrelenting allergies and how badly they were affecting me. She told me something shocking. Before talking with her, I didn't realize how closely our diets affect our health. She had just started working with a health company who worked with NASA to create the Astroade for astronauts to drink on their space missions. I had never even HEARD of some of the things she told me. I learned so much about health from that conversation with her, for example, that milk causes inflammation and thick mucus. How could that be? I loved milk! I drank a gallon of milk every few days. I had no idea. Could I be causing my own health problems?

I decided then that things needed to change.

So I decided to give her advice a shot. After all, if all of this really is backed by science and came with a 100% feel-better guarantee, what did I have to lose? I decided to make some simple diet changes, like giving up sweet tea entirely and replacing it with water. Small changes like this and incorporating more vegetables seemed like it was really turning my health around. I was starting to feel more energized and more alive!

But then I got another sinus infection.

The most serious infection I've ever had in my life. So I met with my friend again to ask how I could finally beat these allergies once and for all. Was it possible to do that without any creepy chemicals or more pharmaceutical prescriptions that didn't work? My journey to health and well-being took more education. My friend gave me some audio recordings to listen to and I learned so much about *feeding* my body nutrients from whole foods. That information really struck me. I decided to try some of her company's products, starting with a multivitamin, alfalfa, and a protein shake. I seriously retooled my diet, starting with eliminating dairy, caffeine, and sugar, *especially* when I was feeling like I was getting sick.

My allergies became manageable for the first time in my life. In fact, I rarely get sinus infections anymore! I've only been on antibiotics five times in the last 25 years. Those few times were when I was under a *lot* of stress. Changing my diet and taking control of my nutrition was the first step of my journey. For example, one of those health flare-ups was when I was preparing to go to Russia to adopt my first child. I always wanted to adopt children not because I couldn't have children, but because there was a deep desire planted in me to do so. I like to say it was a calling from God. But this caused a lot of stress between my husband and me because I desperately wanted to be a stay-at-home mom, but my husband wouldn't allow it. I resigned myself to doing things his way, but his lack of support left me feeling very frustrated.

Luckily, my first daughter came into my life just at the right moment. Veronica was seven years old when she came to live with us and she brought me joy and happiness that was missing from my life.

Eventually, my daughter began to ask for a little sister. I didn't see how that would be possible, since I had spent my entire life savings to adopt her. But I began to pray every night, "God, please provide a way to bring me another daughter and a little sister for Veronica." The thought of the financial burden was stressful for me, but I desperately wanted the best for my little girl. Thankfully, I received a letter from our adoption agency not too long afterwards. The letter was soliciting donations for a new scholarship fund they were creating to help families adopt children with special needs.

I called them and said, "I'm not able to donate at this time but I'm interested in becoming a recipient of the scholarship." Without pause, she said, "I know the perfect child for your family. Her name is Angelica. Let me send you some information." About nine months later, we welcomed our second daughter, seven-year-old Angelica to our family, and all of the expenses for the adoption had been paid in full with the scholarship. I was so grateful that I made a goal to pay it forward in the future.

I couldn't bear the idea of having babies and putting them in day-care, but being able to take my children to school with me and to see them throughout the day was a good enough compromise. Well, for a while at least.

But then it finally happened. After a few years of teaching and parenting, I realized I wasn't giving my best self to my students *or* my children. My voice was so weak when I came home every night, I couldn't even read a story to my children. It definitely wasn't better in the classroom.

I was tired of feeling stressed and depressed every day. I had come too far from where I started to feel like this again. Something had to change.

That's when I decided to build my own business. I wanted to take my destiny into my own hands. I wanted to be able to spend more time with my children and work the hours that fit into my schedule. I decided to partner with the natural nutrition company my friend had recommended, the Shaklee Corporation, because I was so impressed by them. They partner with Nobel Prize winners to innovate new products. Even Olympic athletes trust the products enough to use them. The product ingredients go through a screening process that typically surpasses even the pharmaceutical standards of the US Pharmacopeia. And, they have an income opportunity for people who use and share the products with others. But most important to me are the results I experienced in my own health.

I had struggled with allergies my entire life. No doctor could relieve me of the discomfort and I was finally able to take control of my health with the Shaklee products. I loved the community, support, and instant camaraderie. My skills as a teacher came in handy and helped me to quickly build a business that replaced my salary. I'd found a way to be financially rewarded for helping others create healthier lives. I left my career, my stress was down, and everything really seemed like it was on the way up.

At least it was until my husband (at the time) ran his business into the ground and got us BURIED in debt. The failure was so hard on him, he became unable to work. To support my family, in addition to running my business, I would have to get a corporate job. I needed to replace my husband's salary, but I wasn't about to give up my own dream because of him. I loved the amazing people I'd been able to meet through my business.

The years where I worked two full-time jobs were dark. I had taken a job in corporate wellness. I was the sickest I have ever been in my life. I was living under chronic stress both at work and at home. I found myself in a work environment of lies, betrayal, and back-stabbing. It was taking a toll on me and I knew I couldn't continue like this much longer. If I didn't get my health under control, my health would fail under this high-level stress. I absolutely couldn't let that happen after I had accomplished so much so far. I met my goals in my business, despite having the burden of a second full-time job, and my two daughters had grown up beautifully and graduated high school. I knew something had to change. It was time I took care of myself.

So I quit the job.

I left the toxic marriage.

I moved to a community that was committed to health and wellness.

I began to rebuild my life.

I took a much needed year to heal. I practiced yoga, I walked every day, I took ballroom dancing classes, I learned shuffleboard. I even became a certified health coach! I joined organizations like Rotary, the Chamber of Commerce, and the Holistic Network of Florida. I was doing all of the things I never felt I was able to in my marriage. I surrounded myself with so many positive people; people who were passionate and dedicated to improving themselves. All of this energy was helping me attract the right clients and team members. My business was booming! I finally felt like myself. I was healing emotionally and physically. Most importantly, I was finally able to get my stress under control. That was the key to fully overcoming my chronic health issues.

During my healing, I began to reflect on the lessons I learned.

First, I learned that I was not a victim. I could choose how I eat, think, and live. I could take control of my income and create financial security. Each of my choices would manifest something amazing in my life. I started making healthier choices, such as eliminating toxins in my household cleaners, eating nutritious fruits and vegetables, taking high-quality, natural food-based supplements, and drinking only filtered water. Those were easy changes to make.

Then, the hard choices came, like deciding to find a way to make a living that would allow me time and energy to take care of myself and how to end a marriage of 28 years. But, I am so thankful for the supportive community of people that surrounded me and encouraged me when I made those difficult choices. Otherwise, I would have been stuck in that sick, depressed, and chronically stressed state.

But being strong enough to make those tough choices allowed me to create a business I truly love with my whole heart. I was able to leave a career that was sucking me dry. Today, I have the freedom to dedicate my life to teaching people how to make smart choices for wealth, wellness, and well-being. I build communities online, as well as locally to help people change their lives and become healthier. For example, I run a monthly five-day health reset challenge in a Facebook group, where we commit to five healthy habits for the week: sleep, hydration, inspiration, nutrition, and exercise. Each month, I see lives literally transformed as the participants take time out to practice self-care. It's truly amazing!

So where am I now?

I am living a healthy life in the beautiful city of St. Petersburg, Florida. If you're in St. Petersburg or Tampa Bay, reach out to me! I would love to meet you too. I get to spend each and every day helping people like me. My life's work as I build my Shaklee team is to empower women to make smart choices leading to better health and financial freedom. I know there are many women out there who may feel trapped in situations like I was, whether buried in a mountain of debt, stuck in a low-paying job, trapped in an abusive relationship, or just feeling unfulfilled. And there is a special little place in my heart for the women who want to stay at home with their babies but want to create an income so they can contribute to the family finances. By empowering women with their own business, they can create time freedom and financial freedom. The more people I help, the more value I put out there into the world, and the more I will be rewarded, allowing me to give back even more. My goal now is to reach a level where I can sponsor one adoption scholarship per year!

And if I can do it, you can do it too. Even if you feel stuck, you have the strength inside you to change your whole life too. Never forget it!

"The best way to predict the future is to create it." - *Dr. Forrest Shaklee*

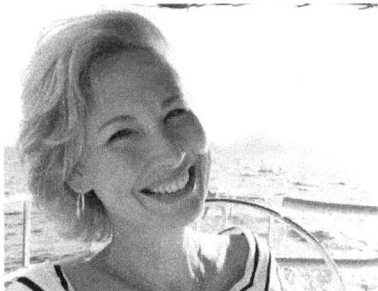

I'm the Wellness Lady. I love empowering people to make smart choices for wealth, wellness, and well-being. I'm passionate about helping people like me who feel like they're stuck in life.

I want you to know that if you're unhappy, you have the strength inside to change. You can build a supportive community around you who you can help. Giving value to a community creates the opportunity for income. If you want some business advice or need support, please email me! I would love to work with you and help you on your journey.

You can transform your life too.

Carla Clayton, Owner of Wellness Lady
Certified Health Coach and Shaklee Independent Distributor
Carla@WellnessLady.com
www.CarlaClayton.com

CHAPTER 6

LIFE RE-IMAGINED

by Clayton Sizemore, Certified Yoga Instructor, RYS 200, Travel
Professional

Former CNN Operations Manager, Clayton Sizemore, returns from India
with a new lease on life.

By today's standards, a 36-year career in a single industry is remarkable.
Longevity and loyalty are often seen as old-fashioned ideals, a reflection of
slower and simpler times in the work world. But for me, 36 years in the
television news industry were filled with satisfaction, success, and
achievement. My first job in TV was an ENG (Electronic News Gathering)
photographer for a local TV station in New Haven, Connecticut, back
when news stories were shot on 16 millimeter film. And now, all of my hard
work and experience in covering and coordinating the logistics surrounding
major news events had advanced me to become the Director of Operations
for CNN New York. Throughout my entire career in broadcasting, I can
truly say I never had a bad day at work. Now, don't get me wrong. There
were challenges, difficult people to work with, and of course the office
politics. But, the thrill of managing reporters, photographers, editors, and
producers was like a drug. No two days were ever the same. Despite all the
things I loved during my later years in the business, I began to experience
the first hints of discontentment and doubt. Where was I going? What was
I doing with my life? The industry I loved and served faithfully was

changing and so was I. As I began to reevaluate, it dawned on me that something was out of balance. I didn't fully understand where this nagging sense of disharmony would lead me. But, it was clear that I needed to identify what I wanted most out of life and set the course for its next phase.

The seed had been planted and the thought of leaving my career behind stirred up all kinds of emotions: anxiety, fear, and uncertainty. But, I was ready to take a leap of faith into the unknown. At the age of 58, I was a widowed father of three incredible adults, an empty nester on my own, living an active and healthy lifestyle. But, with age I found it more challenging to eat right, exercise, manage a demanding work schedule, and take care of my personal life. Something needed to change. I knew that whatever I did next would need to support all of those things and allow me to do good for others as well.

During this time in my life, many men I knew were facing various medical conditions; everything from back issues to high blood pressure to diabetes to cancer. The more research I conducted on good health practices, the more I learned that daily exercise and a healthy diet are the two best things one can embrace in order to stay fit and prolong life. However, at my age weight lifting, marathon training, and the occasional pickup basketball game were not activities I wanted to do or could sustain daily. Yet, these are often the forms of exercise men of my generation, the baby boomers, knew best. And at this age, those practices can sometimes do more harm than good. For these reasons and more, I was pleased to discover yoga.

Yoga. Not what you expected, right? Here I am, a born and bred New York tough guy in my late 50s becoming a yogi. It changed my life. Yoga can enhance every aspect of health – from physical, mental, and emotional to the way we eat. It just made sense. My thoughts were clearer; my body was stronger. I was becoming more mindful and I was definitely more focused. As I benefited more and more from yoga, I knew that I had to share these experiences. I decided to introduce my practice to a group of friends and started what I called, The Men's Movement Class. Designed for men over 50, the focus was on gentle, restorative workouts to tone the body, create strong core muscles, improve flexibility, and strengthen the heart. The class was a success and even men in their 20s and 30s loved it too. I realized that the simplified basic yoga asanas I used were changing the students' perception of exercise and health. That's when I knew to take my leap of faith.

I was an "old school" broadcast journalist ready and willing to do whatever it took to get the job done. To me, it was always about getting the story right. But the industry was changing. Spin, ego, and sensationalism have become key drivers in the broadcast news industry today. I was watching many new people in the business and some seasoned broadcasters make decisions designed to pull in the most viewers, even if it meant focusing on all the wrong things, distorting the truth and addressing self-serving agendas. As a manager, I found myself slowly becoming more of a psychologist, catering to millennials, who lacked the old school values I strongly believed in. Enough was enough and life was calling me in another direction. I wanted to impact my community and others in a more meaningful way. The more I practiced yoga and experienced the benefits of healthy living, the more I became unable and unwilling to settle for a lifestyle and career that I no longer found fulfilling. I started to develop my exit plan from corporate America. After six to eight months of anxiety and second-guessing myself, counseling from friends and family, and a lot of prayer, I was able to walk away from my high-paying job to embrace my new passion.

The first thing I did after leaving CNN was travel to Mysore, India for a 36-day intensive Hatha Yoga teacher training program. It was an experience of a lifetime. Mysore is a strange mix of India's ancient past and its modern state. The city is well-known for its heritage, education, arts, food festivals, ancient temples, and ecology. Mysore is also known as the yoga capital of southern India.

The Ayur Yoga Eco Ashram (www.ayuryoga-ashram.com) in Mysore, India is a first-class operation that focuses on the total yoga experience. Literally, ashram means a place where a group of people live and work together with a common goal of spiritual growth and self-realization. Going to an ashram can help others recharge their spiritual batteries, away from all the distractions of a busy and materialistic lifestyle in society.

Hatha yoga is the most widely practiced form of yoga in America. It focuses on physical health and well-being using bodily postures (asana), breathing techniques (pranayama), and meditation; with the goal of bringing about a sound, healthy body, and a clear, peaceful mind. Students of Hatha yoga are convinced of its power to build strength and confidence, to improve flexibility, and to balance and foster spiritual peace and contentment. Research has shown that yoga can minimize hypertension, strengthen bones, and keep excess pounds at bay. Many also believe in the power of yoga to aid in recovery from everything from back problems to carpel tunnel syndrome, and to help people cope with chronic problems, such as arthritis, multiple sclerosis, and infections.

Here's a look at my daily practice at the ashram in Mysore:

- 5:30 a.m., a 30 to 40-minute meditation
- 7:00 a.m. to 9:00 a.m., practice yoga asanas
- 9:15 a.m., a traditional Indian vegetarian brunch
- 10:30 a.m. to 12:30 p.m., yoga theory classes
- 12:30 p.m. to 2:00 p.m., private coaching or nap time (my favorite)
- 2:30 p.m. to 4:00 p.m., more yoga theory classes
- 4:30 p.m. to 7:00 p.m., teacher training yoga practice
- 7:15 p.m., a traditional Indian vegetarian dinner
- 8:00 p.m. to 9:00 p.m., more classes on anatomy followed by bedtime

It was an extremely regimented and truly life-changing experience. I could see and feel the changes as the days passed; my body was getting stronger and my mind clearer.

From a yogic perspective, people are pressured and even brainwashed to lead a robotic lifestyle, which can be shallow and sometimes meaningless. Being in the ashram helped challenge my own beliefs and values that guided my lifestyle for far too long. Secluded and surrounded by the energy of like-minded people, I was able to combat compulsive behaviors, negative attitude, bad habits, and stressful obligations. At an ashram, we dare to ask: *What am I doing with my life? Why? What do I really want? And how can I live a purposeful and fulfilling life?* At the end of my time in Mysore, I was not only able answer these questions, but to practice the techniques that I needed to reset my body and mind for a fresh start. It was what I needed to reimagine my life.

The meaning of yoga is to unite and after a month of daily meditation, yoga practice, theory, teacher training, and a strict vegetarian diet, I was ready to come home and take my experience and new-found knowledge to the next level with the Urban Yoga Foundation (www.urbanyogafoundation.org). The Urban Yoga Foundation (UYF) is a nonprofit organization that educates and empowers communities to be proactive about issues affecting their health. Through yoga and related holistic approaches, UYF programs help individuals manage stress, develop mind-body awareness, and health consciousness. For 20-years, UYF has continued its important work of designing health programs throughout the greater New York area and now in St Petersburg, Florida. We provide yoga and mindfulness courses to companies and institutions seeking to create a productive, innovative, healthy, and harmonious environment. Our development workshops incorporate various exercises involving simple, stress-relieving postures, meditation, breath work, and other positive tools to help employees manage and mitigate stress. Program length, dates, frequency, and content can be customized to serve your specific needs and interest.

The Men's Movement class now has a certified yoga instructor…me! And when I look back on all of this, I am humbled and proud to say that trusting my feelings and keeping my faith made all the difference in the world. Leaving a secure work environment and a comfortable way of life after so many years was one of the hardest things I have ever done. But what I learned has been more than worth the cost. As we chase life and seek to find fulfillment and our calling, sometimes we have to step outside our comfort zone and take that risk. It can be scary, but fear is the opposite of faith. Blessings and Namaste!

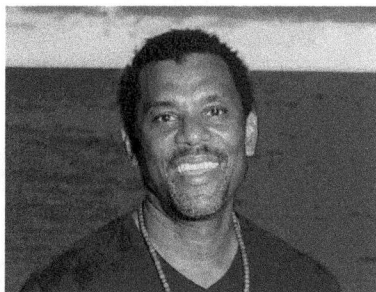

After 36 years as a broadcast manager working for ABC, NBC, and the world news leader CNN, Sizemore has re-imagined his career by taking control of his future, embarking on the next phase of chasing life and longevity as a certified yoga instructor and certified Paycation travel agent.

Born in Mount Vernon, New York, Sizemore grew up in an environment of social empowerment and change. Personal childhood influences from leaders in politics, arts, and religion like Nina Simone, Betty Shabazz, Adam 'Clayton' Powell, and Langston Hughes all made impressions. Those impressions set a standard for excellence that remains a part of his personal and professional work ethic.

A resident of St Petersburg Florida, Sizemore is a partner and senior instructor at the Urban Yoga Foundation and the father of three amazing adults. Clayton Sizemore believes that with faith, all things are possible!

Clayton Sizemore, Certified Yoga Instructor, RYS 200, Travel Professional
sizemore0@aol.com
www.urbanyogafoundation.org
www.speakeasytravel.paycation.com
908-721-2362

CHAPTER 7

THE HEALING ROAD
by Kimberly Dixson, Wholistic Health Coach, Yoga Instructor,
Chinese Herbalist

If you asked me one year ago if I thought I would have a life as a thriving, sober health coach, I would have shrugged "meh" and poured myself another glass of wine. You just may have to use your coping skills for the next few paragraphs.

I had to muster up daily phony smiles through one of the most painful separations of my life. I was being forced to move because I was no longer welcome to share a life with the person I moved 700 miles to be with. I was stuck in the middle of suburbia NC with no friends. I sobbed (hard) through three different jobs, double shifts, long hours I could not stand, just to make enough money to move. I started a GoFundMe account just to be able to purchase a bicycle to ride. I put myself through every online video assignment of "eat well and feel good!!" when I was going through anything BUT that. I was also helping myself to about one to two bottles of wine a night and fighting the daily physical ache of losing everything I dreamed, hoped, and cared for in a matter of dwindling weeks. Time felt like a ticking bomb.

It was clear to me I was hot mess but ready or not, I was being prepped to transform.

It is impossible to teach this kind of deep transformation to anyone because it is such an innate, raw, hard core experience that shakes you to your soul; and I mean literally shook me in a panic. I would wake from awful dreams in tears and just needing HIM or some THING to hold on to. Maybe he will change his mind and not want to break it off? Maybe I'm not cut out for this "health coach" thing? What is this hopeless search for internal happiness that everyone says is inside each of us?

I knew my path was going to never be carved, paved, or made easy for me since a young age. My life as I knew it so far was full of painful experience, deceitful relationships, abandonment, living the "nobody gets me" victim role. But there was some really great stuff, too…and I could see it was all forming me, somehow.

I was aware through many teachings, lectures, books and gurus that perhaps I chose these particularly awesome experiences. I had driven across countries and moved over oceans on my own, on barely 500 dollars in my pocket each time. I've been so lucky to experience some of the most amazing beauty in this world that some may never see in their whole lives. I have put myself through school after school, certification after certification just to make one more notch in my belt, to earn myself some respect. My tattered heart is a brave and courageous one, but it had to be awakened along the way. From doing intakes with women, who have just been raped, then dropped off at my resident safe house by an uncaring cop to a strange place, while having to re-live her gruesome explanation to me; when I shared in cooking Thanksgiving dinner for a house full of schizophrenics at the mental facility I worked at because their families would never acknowledge their existence ever again; when I would teach weekly yoga to the aging senior doing everything she could to get to every single one of my classes because her dignity and deep rooted heritage of Ohana and Aloha was far more important to her than whatever she looked like doing the poses…these are the courageous humans I have been so lucky to learn from. They have touched my life and I know that I have touched theirs.

Fast forward to today, honoring my own story gives people permission to live theirs and vice versa.

I am consistently tapping my intuition when helping today's clients, whether it be toward better education on food choices, daily sobriety, having a friendly ear to bend, or a meaningful embrace. Reading people's internal stuff has never been difficult for me. Having grown up quickly in an alcoholic broken family and being continuously exposed to abuse makes your intuition pretty sharp. Discovering this gave me a special understanding of clients; a certain perspective. Even up to this day in my advanced schooling, with my friendships, and my employment status; I knew that until I was going to make the decisions with the conviction I needed to, unless I made it a MUST, I was going to feel like a fraud. I had to rescue my own shine so that maybe I could provide some light for anyone else traveling in that similar darkness. I was willing to accept it was my own head that created those opinions about my worth. I was willing to accept my painful past with equanimity, and forgive even silently the people I have felt I was wronged by...even when it didn't feel that I could. My life's passion is to let people know I have been there. I understand. I recognize that you are a rare experience to be shared.

Aaaand (haha) then again, some people just want to know exactly what healthy foods to eat. That is also VERY OK! It's surprising to some that health coaching is not only about the food. Eventually, they come around full circle to find it goes so much deeper than that. Ahhh, if only one's true motivation for life were found in a crown of broccoli...

I find deep healing recovery through food and color vibration. I truly believe in the power of your relationship to fresh, wholesome, living foods that aren't abusive to your body, and tapping an energy outlet conducive to your physicality; also not one that beats up your body. Open to healing herbs, we explore western and eastern herbal plants and a host of other alkalizing tools that may help fill some of the potholes on the healing road. Because THAT is what we are here to do...create our own path, cut through the thicket, end the excuses, and discover the secrets to our passion. So, WHAT FULFILLS YOU? What sustains and motivates each person to say, *enough-is-enough, I'm ready for a change*? Where have you set the bar on your own standards, peaks, and valleys? Are you ready to say, *so what if you mess it up but go big anyway*?

What do you think of when you hear "change" and "transformation?" The words sound so lively, exciting, thrilling to some and downright frightful for others. Some live unhappily in the safety, rather than step fully into their greatness because they may not know what that even looks like. They can eat all of the kale in the world, but that will not change the fact they stay with a partner who is abusive and thoughtless. To live in this cycle means stress is driving, cortisol is pumping like gasoline, unable to lose the weight, brain fog gets worse...so the vicious cycle of fear continues. Most people are so used to the duress they are living. They don't see it as a struggle. They view CHANGE as the struggle; the harder path, the more difficult choice. Living in fulfillment isn't something you have to give up or constantly force yourself to have positive thoughts about. It takes dedication to finding what satisfies the bigger vision. It takes forethought AND risk. It takes planning AND a leap of faith. They meet as one path, not in opposition of each other. They are partnered to help shape one's destiny.

As for me, my life (as I knew it) was a falling tower, whether I liked it or not, one year ago today. I did move back to St. Petersburg and was welcomed back. I graduated from the nutrition program, I stopped the wine medicating, I dropped the weight, and I buried the decayed relationship that I was hanging on to for dear life. I've gained a number of clients within the very first month of graduation. I have had the most wonderful conversations in and out of my business each day. I ran two half marathons, rode a solo metric century bike ride, joined more social events, practiced yoga again, and I hold my own spiritual ceremonies. I began a Chinese Herbalist program. I feel open to new experiences every day I step into work. I acknowledge my worth, my growth, and my creativity. I wrote this chapter, as it's been a life-long dream to be published. I'm taking that trip I've dreamed up for so long. I can literally feel the love the Universe is providing for me. I can finally say I trust my spirit guides are working in my favor. I believe it IS very much a conspiracy that the best of your lessons are at work for you. It's all about the leap inside. Take one full, deep breath at a time. Step off into your joy. Say good riddance to fear with clear-headed, open-hearted goodness.

You have so got this!

Love and Light

42

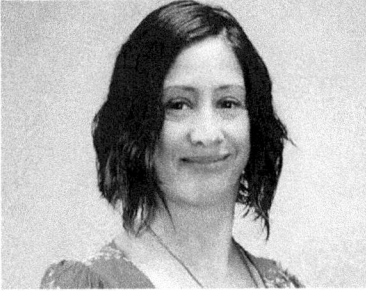

Wholistic Health Coach, Kimberly Dixson completed her training at the Institute for Integrative Nutrition, where she studied a variety of dietary theories and practical lifestyle coaching methods. Kimberly has completed extensive studies and practices for over 15 years in the world of whole food nutrition, vitamins, herbal supplements, yoga, and alternative healing methods. With many years in the health field, Kimberly has helped thousands of students, customers, and clients get in touch with their life, and works personally one-on-one with clients on a monthly basis, and also through Rollin Oats Market as a supplement specialist.

Kimberly Dixson, Wholistic Health Coach, Yoga Instructor, Chinese Herbalist
binka117@yahoo.com
www.facebook.com/WholisticCoachKim

HOLISTIC APPROACH

CHAPTER 8

FARM OVER PHARMA

by Vanessa Sardi, MS, CHE, CHC

I'm a 40-year-old Cardiovascular Physiologist, Certified Health & Nutrition Coach, who was born and raised in New Orleans, Louisiana. As a former cheerleader for the NFL Saints, you might say I'm a 'Who Dat' fan! I love to travel, dance, read, spend time with my dogs, play the piano, and I LOVE the beach. I am a recovering anorexic and bulimic - November 2017 will mark 11 years in recovery! Needless to say, I had an extremely unhealthy relationship with food for most of my life. Now, food is my friend. It is the nourishment for my mind, body, and soul. And when I'm sick (which I can't remember the last time I was), it's my "go-to" medicine.

I am at my absolute happiest when I am helping others, whether that's helping them to change their lifestyle, lose unwanted weight, reverse their disease, offering hope to those still suffering in the grips of addiction, or encouraging those who are on their journey to becoming the healthiest version of themselves. I had such a blast cheering in the NFL and now I want to be YOUR biggest cheerleader!

I spent the first five years of my career out of graduate school working as a cardiopulmonary physiologist. You might ask, what the heck does that mean? I designed exercise rehabilitation programs for heart and lung disease patients. I worked predominately with elderly people who soon became my second family. I absolutely adored my patients! They were very special to me and there's nothing I wouldn't have done for them. I am the person I am today because of the life lessons I learned from these very wise people. They will always have a special place in my heart.

In 2004, the physicians who owned the cardiopulmonary rehabilitation center were being forced to close the clinic due to changes in Medicare reimbursement. They were losing money and therefore, had to make the very difficult decision to shut down. My first thought was, *What were my patients going to do? Who was going to take care of them like I did?* Then, it dawned on me, in two weeks, I was going to be out of a job!

It was nothing short of a blessing when I was offered a position as a sales representative for one of the largest pharmaceutical companies in the world. During my nine years as a rep, I sold multiple medications to almost every type of specialist in multiple disease markets: men's health, women's health, ENTs, pediatrics, internal medicine, endocrinology, and cardiology to name a few. Throughout my career as a rep, I believed WHOLE-HEARTEDLY that I was doing the right thing for patients. I couldn't have promoted products I didn't believe in because a salesman I was NOT. What I didn't realize at the time was, I was being brainwashed by "big pharma." They did an EXCELLENT job convincing their reps we were "saving patient's lives" by the work we did every day. Today, I realize more pills doesn't translate to better health. In fact, it's just the opposite!

When I left big pharma, I went to work for a small, private company that specializes in cardiovascular genomics. My call points were primary care physicians and cardiologists. Indeed, this was much more in alignment with my morals, both as a professional and as a human being. Then one day, I watched a documentary on Netflix that would change my life forever entitled, *Forks Over Knives*. This led me to multiple nutrition conferences all over the U.S., including our capitol, Washington, D.C., where I got to meet and speak with the former president of the American College of Cardiology. He is a wonderful man who understands the many benefits of a whole food, plant-based diet and follows one too! I got to meet Dr. Caldwell Esselstyn, Cleveland Clinic, T. Collin Campbell, PhD, Cornell University, Dr. Dean Ornish, who helped President Bill Clinton adopt a whole food, plant-based diet after his bypass surgery, and Dr. Pam Popper, CEO of Wellness Forum. I became obsessed with researching and learning as much as possible about nutrition and its role in disease reversal and disease prevention. Before I knew it, I was back in school to become certified in plant-based nutrition by Cornell University.

Now that I knew beyond any shadow of a doubt, a whole food, plant-based lifestyle could reverse coronary artery disease, I began asking cardiologists what they were doing to help patients change their diets. I was flabbergasted when 99% of them told me they were doing NOTHING! I could've gotten angry. However, I knew doctors received zero nutrition training in medical school. What angered me was that none of them believed in their patients' ability to make lifestyle changes. They would tell me, "Vanessa, they aren't going to change the way they eat. So, why even bother?" I EVEN HAD ONE CARDIOLOGIST TELL ME, "Seeing patients in clinic is boring. I'd much rather take people to the cath lab to do angiograms. Those are way more exciting." In other words, people were having invasive procedures they didn't need to have, that didn't come without risk and discomfort to the patient, as well as a 1% mortality rate!

I spent a lot of time in Cardiology because I sold cardiovascular medication, as well as a diagnostic test to detect the presence and extend of obstructive coronary artery disease. I learned a lot about business acumen, the reimbursement system, managed care, and what motivates both doctors and insurance companies to make the decisions they make regarding a patient's care. Unfortunately, those decisions aren't always driven by what's best for the patient. This isn't to say doctors are bad people. Many of them are very good people, operating in a very corrupt healthcare (or more appropriately, "disease-care") system.

Cardiologists perform nuclear stress tests to uncover any blockages a patient may have in their coronary vessels. It was one of many diagnostic tools used to assess heart disease. This diagnostic tool is intended for high-risk, symptomatic patients. However, I witnessed cardiologists ordering it like routine testing in patients who were low risk and 100% asymptomatic.

A nuclear stress test measures blood flow to your heart during rest and while your heart is working harder (stressed), due to either exertion or medication that induces stress. If you've never had one, they take anywhere from two to four hours and they aren't much fun. The drugs they use dilate the arteries of the heart and increase blood flow to help show any blockages or obstructions in the heart's arteries.

One of the issues with this test is its inability to detect "bilateral ischemia." Meaning, if you have equivalent or close to equivalent blockages on BOTH sides of your heart, your nuclear scan will look normal. There has to be an IMBALANCE for an abnormality to show. People who have significant blockages on both sides of their heart are ticking time bombs. They're the ones told they have a normal stress test, then go home the next day and die of a massive heart attack, leaving everyone scratching their heads wondering what the heck happened!

Let's talk radiation exposure. International law states that any healthcare provider working in nuclear medicine cannot be exposed to more than 20 mSv (miliseiverts - a biological measurement) of radiation per year because radiation is cumulative. That's why you see all of them wearing a little monitor on their scrubs. One study stated, for every additional 10 millisieverts (mSv) in cumulative radiation dose received, the risk of developing cancer rose by three percent.[1]

We're exposed to radiation every day in our normal environment. However, the diagnostic tools in the medical field, particularly the nuclear scan and the PET/CT scan, expose people to more radiation than anything else; except for the Hiroshima bomb! One cardiac nuclear stress test exposes a patient to up to 40 mSv of radiation…just ONE test! [3][4] That far exceeds the amount that is allowed for healthcare professionals working in that field! What about the patients? One cardiac nuclear stress test is the radiation equivalent of 500-600 chest x-rays at one time!!

The definition of informed consent is "permission granted in the knowledge of the possible consequences, typically that which is given by a patient to a doctor for treatment with full knowledge of the possible risks and benefits." Unfortunately, in my experience, that rarely happened. It's your right to ask your doctor if the risks outweigh the benefits for any test, procedure or drug. Ask how much radiation you are being exposed to for any given diagnostic test; ask if there is an alternative diagnostic test they can run that poses fewer side effects…ask ask ask! You deserve the right to know exactly what is going into your body, the benefits, and most importantly, the consequences!

The driving force behind what I do is educate people because the more people know, the better decisions they are able to make regarding their health. We SHOULD NOT be nodding "yes" to every prescription pill, diagnostic test, and procedure our doctors order for us. I'm not saying doctors are bad people at all. They are simply doing what they were taught to do in medical school…treat symptoms and diseases rather than the underlying cause of disease. My passion and my goal is to help people lose weight without diet pills, calorie counting, or calorie restriction; to help people PREVENT AND REVERSE DISEASE using FOOD AS MEDICINE, while living a life of compassion for ourselves, one another, our planet and all sentient beings!

The top three killers in the U.S. are heart disease, cancer, and medical error. Based on an analysis of prior research, the Johns Hopkins study estimates that more than 250,000 Americans die each year from medical errors. On the CDC's official list, that would rank just behind heart disease and cancer, which each took about 600,000 lives in 2014, and in front of respiratory disease, which caused about 150,000 deaths.[4] All three of these diseases are preventable! Most of the westernized diseases we see today (heart disease, cancer, type 2 diabetes, and autoimmune diseases) are diseases of lifestyle. This means if lifestyle got people into this mess, then lifestyle will get people out of this mess. What you choose to fuel your body with is one of the most important decisions you can possibly make for yourself. You can literally eat your way into or out of disease! With every bite of food you take, you are either promoting wellness or contributing to illness. It only takes one unhealthy meal comprised of processed foods and animal products to cause inflammation inside your coronary vessels. And it takes approximately six hours for your body to return to normal, which it's then time for lunch or dinner!

I cannot emphasize enough how important it is to add more fruits, vegetables, whole grains, and beans into your meal plan. I have watched people completely reverse type 2 diabetes and discontinue all their medication by consuming a whole food, plant-based diet. I have watched people with Crohn's disease, lupus, psoriasis, Celiac, rheumatoid arthritis, restless leg syndrome, and more go into remission by following a whole food, plant-based diet. I have a friend who had stage 4 metastatic breast cancer who became cancer free simply by changing what she ate. Will this happen for everyone? Who knows. But what I do know is that while there are hundreds of pills to treat just one disease state, there is one diet that halts and reverses most chronic conditions we see today. It really is that simple!

1. www.cmaj.ca/content/early/2011/02/07/cmaj.100463.abstract
2. hps.org/documents/meddiagimaging.pdf
3. www.health.harvard.edu/cancer/radiation-risk-from-medical-imaging
4. www.npr.org/sections/health-shots/2016/05/03/476636183/death-certificates-undercount-toll-of-medical-errors

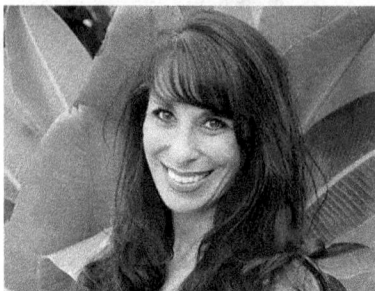

Vanessa is a certified health and nutrition coach with a unique perspective on health and wellness. She has a master's degree in Cardiopulmonary Physiology, a bachelor's degree in Sports Medicine, clinical work in cardiopulmonary rehabilitation, and research/sales experience in pharmaceutical and gene expression testing. Vanessa has a passion for nutrition and helping others to live healthy, fueled by her background and consistent studies. When Vanessa realized that "more pills" wasn't the answer to better health, she walked away from her job at one of the largest pharmaceutical companies in the world to start her own business, Nutriception.

Vanessa Sardi, MS, CHE, CHC
vanessa@nutriception.net
www.nutriception.net
facebook.com/FARMoverPHARMA
219-237-8466

CHAPTER 9

HEALING FROM HEARTACHE AND LEARNING TO LOVE MYSELF

by Anne Dort, Certified Clinical and Family Herbalist, Holistic Health Coach

Anyone who has ever suffered any kind of heartache knows just how much it can weaken your immune system making you more susceptible to illness and the effects it has on your mental and emotional health. Typically, self-care goes out the window at least in the beginning of a heart break/heart ache, which definitely takes a toll on the body, mind, and spirit. Did you know, according to the Harvard Medical School and the Mayo Clinic, suffering from heartache puts you at a much higher risk for heart attack and "Broken Heart Syndrome?" Yes, "Broken Heart" is an actual medical diagnosis. This is just one of the many reasons why it is absolutely vital to provide unconditional love and compassion for yourself at all times. In this chapter, you will learn how I healed from major heartache and learned to love myself. I hope that my journey will serve as a resource of tools to help ease the symptoms of heart break for someone else.

The common misperception is that putting your needs and desires first or ahead of anyone else is selfish. According to the Merriam Webster dictionary, the definition of "selfish" is "concerned excessively or exclusively with oneself; seeking or concentrating on one's own advantage, pleasure, or well-being without regard for others." If you are a mother or a caregiver, forget about it. How dare you? Let the shaming and guilt begin. Please hear me on this. We have got it all wrong. Unless you completely disregard the well-being of others, loving yourself and self-love do not, I repeat, do not equate to being selfish. You cannot love your neighbor as you love yourself, if you do not love yourself in the first place. You cannot be of service to others if you do not take care of yourself.

What if the importance of loving ourselves could be ingrained early on in childhood and we could do away with the fantasy "someday your prince will come and love you and you'll live happily ever after.?" It should be as important as learning to love your family, or as a part of personal hygiene, so to say. If we could teach this early on, then our children, confidently knowing their self-worth, would be able to start off creating healthy boundaries socially; thereby potentially avoiding misguided choices and painful mistakes commonly made in our younger years, and weaken the blows of inevitable heartache.

Unfortunately for most of us, the importance of self-love is learned much later on in life. Typically, after we hit rock bottom is when we wake up. It may take someone or something lovingly shaking us to snap out of it and come to our own rescue. A job loss, deadly addiction, an unexpected death, sudden illness, serious accident, disaster, a big move, a breakup, separation, all forms of domestic violence, or divorce can all cause heartache. No one wants to experience these tragic and stressful life situations; most of us will at one point or another. Having the right tools and seeking outside help as needed to navigate this period of time is super crucial for our wellbeing.

For me, the realization came after separation from my marriage of eight years. I had to leave my home suddenly, which meant leaving behind life as I had known it and stepping into the unknown with my children. We left behind memories and belongings and dreams. I left behind friends and responsibilities. I had to start from ground zero with nothing. I felt hopeless and scared and alone inside.

Thankfully, I had my two children, my godson, his pup, and my two best friends of over 20 years by my side keeping me company, so I was never really alone, alone. This became our new family structure. We cooked dinner every night, ate around the dinner table, electronic free, and had conversations about the things that matter in life. We did lots of arts and crafts with the kids and had family dance nights and celebrations. They put up with my medicine making, moon tea, crystals, and sage. I can't find words to express what they did for us. But it was major life support when we needed it the most. I will always and forever be grateful for them.

It wasn't always sunshine and butterflies for me. Underneath all the welcomed distraction, no matter how hard I tried, I still felt alone inside. Thoughts just went round and round in my head. Why was I not worthy of love? Why were the kids not enough of a reason to get help? For the first time, I was seeing everything as it really was and not how I wanted to believe. It was a harsh reality I had chosen not to acknowledge up until this moment.

Between the tears and the prayers, I heard the soothing voice of my inner guide: "You do deserve genuine love and kindness and respect. The reason you have not yet known that kind of love is because you have never in all your life loved and valued yourself. You have always put other's feelings before your own, stifled your voice out of fear, been afraid to shine your light and have been quiet for far too long. You've always been submissive, and physically, socially, and spiritually confined in your relationships. Now is your chance to start fresh, to make a change and stop the pattern you've been stuck in. You must love yourself the way you want to be loved. You have not suffered time after time after time in your relationships in vain. It has been an assignment for you to learn from. It is going to help others to share your story. It is time to acknowledge and heal from traumas of the past, and to love yourself."

And so it began…my mission…"Love Anne"

Emotional support: It is important to identify your support system as early on as possible after a heart ache. Believe me, you are going to need them. Whether it's close family members or your closest friends or a local support group. (Thank you to everyone and anyone that reached out to me, and offered a cup of tea and lent an ear or even just a hug. You know who you are and I thank you from the bottom of my heart.) There are support groups for every kind of situation. You just have to do a little research. I joined a local women's creative arts group (little did I know it was a new group and was starting the very first day I attended.) It has been the best thing I have ever done for myself. The group meets weekly and offers us a chance to share our week and how we are feeling. As we do that, we color or make something symbolic of our journey and our strength. We painted coffee mugs, made mindfulness jars, painted rocks, made collages, had letting go ceremonies, and journaled. The stories of these woman touched my heart. We had all been in the same shoes at one point or another. Even the facilitators Tina and Lola had been in our shoes and had decided to use their journeys out of the darkness to share their light and support with other women like us. Lola, the head facilitator became my biggest cheerleader, a mentor, and a guardian angel. She inspires me so much.

Vision board: The first week I attended the group, we created vision boards. I had no idea we were going to that. I had been wanting to create one, now that life was going to be different and I needed some vision of where I wanted to go in life. And here it was that the opportunity was right before me. My vision board was of living on or near the beach and having an apothecary/wellness center (half of that has since come to pass). Try to envision what you want your future to look like in every area of life. Where are you going? Draw or create a collage of your vision and put it someplace you will see every day.

Journaling: The second week I attended group, we were decorating journals and were encouraged to write in them as much as possible; to "brain dump" everything that was going on in our life at the end of our day; anything that was building up that we needed to get out or things we didn't feel comfortable sharing out loud. It was one of the most instrumental tools during this time and still is. It's amazing to look back and see how far you've come and to honor your journey.

Connecting with nature: As much as you may be tempted to stay curled up inside and in bed, you have to make time to get outside for some vitamin D and getting your hands dirty in the soil is always a plus. I would make a point to get outside at least five minutes daily. It gave me the opportunity to be present in the moment and mindful. A peaceful observer of Mother Nature doing her thing; paying attention to the plants, the spiders delicately spinning their webs, squirrels munching on fresh mushrooms and acorns, bees and butterflies pollinating and suckling nectar. It's really humbling to witness how much goes on all around us that we are too busy to notice. I began talk therapy with an amazing therapist. Thankfully for me, she had a strong connection to nature as well. We would meet in my favorite park. I spilled my heart out to her every week. She gave me wonderful guidance and direction when I couldn't see the forest through the trees. By the end of our talks, I would be giving a "weed walk," identifying and showing her which weeds and plants around us were edible or medicinal. She was not at all afraid to taste the purslane or the beautiful fruiting beauty berries and she was excited to learn.

Bath time is sacred: If you have a bathtub, you have a healing haven. Bath time is a personal weekly healing ritual I started long ago. It's so important to cleanse your energy field and your physical body of toxins we pick up throughout our days and carry with us. The difference between just a nice hot relaxing bath and a healing bath is in super charging the water. Here is my magic recipe: fill the tub with hot/warm water, then add 2-3 cups of Epsom salt, and ¼ to ½ cup of baking soda. From there, you can personalize it as you like. You can add a few drops of lavender essential oil mixed with equal amounts coconut oil into the salt or add a couple drops of flower essences to the water. Light some soy candles and surround yourself with beautiful crystals. I recommend placing some amethyst and rose quartz crystals into the bath water with you. Put on a nice meditation and use this alone time to quiet your mind and connect with your inner guidance. Soak for 20-45 minutes.

Crystals: Crystals emit energy/vibration. They can be used to balance the chakras, for emotional healing, protection, grounding and to attract the energy associated with them. You can hold them while mediating. Use them as decor. Infuse your drinking water or bath water with them and more. When it comes to healing heartache, rose quartz will be your best friend. It facilitates heart healing, self-love, and inner peace. I carried it on me at all times. I would use it to sooth my heartache and clear any blocks I had to love. I would hold it as a reminder to love myself more deeply.

Essential oils: Lavender essential oil is a tool I carry with me everywhere. It promotes a feeling of peace and calm. I can pull it out anytime I need to center myself and stay calm. Open the top and smell right from the bottle to experience the benefits.

Flower essences: Flower energy is very subtle, yet very effective on the emotions. I like to use flower essences from a local herbalist known for her use of Florida blooms. If you can't get a hold of a local organic source, try Bach's Rescue Remedy. Take a drop or two under the tongue in times of stress.

YouTube: In the beginning of my heart ache, feeling alone, I started to wonder if any women like me were blogging their journeys out of the empath/narcissist relationship dynamic. I stumbled across the channel, "Darienne Empire." Darienne's videos on living as an empath and rocking it, and on depression helped get me through this time and taught me a lot about myself that I hadn't realized. Since childhood, I knew I was highly-sensitive. I felt what other people were feeling as if it were happening to me. I never spoke about it to anyone. In my young adult life, I had been taken advantage of numerous times because I was overly empathetic, so finding this was a blessing. I also found out I could connect with her daily as she did live ACIM video lessons on her Facebook page. Her raw authenticity is what I love most about her. She is a fierce and brave woman, not afraid to tell it like it is, and also to share her story to help others. Her adorable baby girl makes a daily appearance; usually to climb up and blow kisses to the camera or hold her mother's crystals. Her beautiful teenage daughter even pops in every once in a while to say hello. She shows us you can rock mom life and not let spiritual life fall by the wayside. Now I am going to be taking her training for empaths. Finding this channel changed my life.

Emotional Freedom Technique: EFT or "tapping" was a useful tool when I felt anxiety and paralyzed by my fears, not wanting to get out of bed. It is a very simple technique to retrain your neural pathways and your amygdala's response to fear. It's helpful with depression and post-traumatic stress and triggers. I highly recommend reading *The Tapping Solution* by Nick Ortner and also watching the documentary, *The Tapping Solution* to learn how to use it for yourself. EFT is also all about learning to love and accept yourself as you are.

Rose water: A dear local herbalist friend of mine, Linda gifted me with her handcrafted organic rose water and rose elixir, and I could not have done without either. Rose is a wonderful plant ally for grieving and for all matters of the energetic heart. Here was my routine: every morning when I woke up, I would stand in front of the mirror and take a dropper full of the rose elixir under my tongue and hold it for a few seconds before swallowing. Next, I would spray my face and then my chest, directly over my heart. I would then place both my hands over my heart and look at myself and say, "I love you Anne. I truly, deeply love you." I would repeat this routine each night before bed as well; sometimes midday too, if I felt the need.

Treat yourself: Buy those flowers you've been waiting for. Buy yourself the jewelry you had hoped for. Take yourself on romantic candle-lit dinner for one, a walk on the beach at sunset, or a stroll around the farmer's market with a cup of local roasted coffee or cup of tea. Start to take responsibility for fulfilling your own desires and for your happiness. Treat yourself the way you want to be treated by someone else.

Nutrition: Each time you go to put something in your mouth, ask yourself "Is this worthy of going into my body? Is this food whole, nourishing and pure or dead and devoid of all real nutritional energy and value? Is this loving my body? Is it truly feeding my body or am I bored or sad or just eating to satisfy a craving?" Magnesium is a wonderful supplement to look into during this time, as well as a good probiotic.

Mindset: This will likely come later on after the initial heartache and the emotional roller coaster that may ensue. You have to come to a place where you will be willing to see things differently. See your fears through eyes of love instead. See your situation as a spiritual assignment. Learn to implement the law of attraction and find or create a sacred space. Connect with your higher power. Prayer is powerful. Start attending temple, church services, spiritual groups, or bible studies. Whatever your beliefs, you can find groups and services online too. Belly breathing, meditation, and Louis Hay affirmations will help tremendously with mindset as well.

These methods of self-love cannot stop once things seem to fall into place and get better. Just like all relationships, your relationship to yourself takes some intentional maintenance. I still do these things on a regular basis as I continue to learn and grow. I hope that you will use this chapter as inspiration to take a leap of faith into the unknown and chase the happiness you deserve, and as a tool box in times of heartache and seasons of change. You are not alone. You will get through this. Take care of yourself and you will see. You got this.

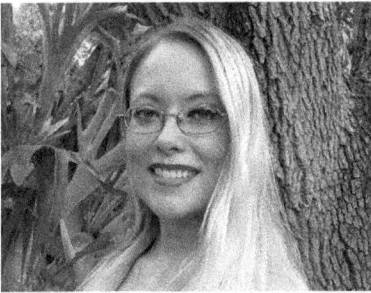

Anne is the owner of Awaken~ Balance~ Transform. She is a certified clinical and family herbalist, owns an herbal product line called, "Herbal Annie's," and is a former president of The Florida Herb Society. She is a holistic health coach, Level II certified Usui Reiki practitioner, and certified crystal healer. Anne is a graduate of the Professional Herbalist Training Program at Acupuncture and Herbal Therapies and has completed Spirit Junkie Masterclass Level 1 training with Gabrielle Bernstein. She is an ordained minister and mom on-the-go.

My mission is to inspire and guide you on an unapologetic journey of self-love and personal transformation, and to empower you to be your greatest resource.

Anne Dort, Certified Clinical and Family Herbalist, Holistic Health Coach
www.awakenbalancetransform.blogspot.com
www.instagram.com/herbalanniesflorida
YouTube: Awaken Balance Transform
www.facebook.com/OrganicElderberrySyrup
awakenbalancetransform@gmail.com
herbalannie2013@gmail.com

CHAPTER 10

WANDERING PATHS
by Lena Roberts, LMT, NMT

Hi. My name is Lena and I am a lot of things... mother, wife, licensed massage therapist, and business owner. More importantly, I am a loving, kind, caring, and compassionate person that takes an interest in helping others feel better. My journey has some early origins to help pique my interest. Like many other people my age, I worked a few jobs along the way to help pay the bills and stay involved, but it wasn't until my kids graduated that I allowed myself to evolve in this direction fully. Here is a little more detail...

Before I was five years old, I encountered an injured dog. His leg was broken and the only time that he would stop whining or yelping in pain is when I was touching it. I realized that my touch was comforting and that I could have an extremely positive impact on other living things through touch.

In the third grade, I had a strep infection. My mom took me to the hospital and told me that everyone there would help me feel better. Being that they were successful in making me feel better, I learned that the hospital was a good place to be if I wanted to help people feel better too.

My friend's grandmother overheard us talking about our summer plans and suggested volunteering at the hospital as a candy striper. A candy striper would do things like push a cart with coffee, snacks, and periodicals to offer the patients. I would also run errands for the nurses, like taking samples to the lab. This sounded like fun and remembering my earlier experiences, was something I wanted to do. I did this for two years and really enjoyed sitting and spending time with people. I really felt like I was making a difference to the patients and their families. On one occasion, I was delivering a sample to the lab at the age of 16 and the director asked if I would like to have a job and get paid. YES! I became a receptionist at the hematology lab. I worked in that capacity for two years until I graduated high school. I was not thrilled in this job. I was in a cubicle and no longer had any real contact with patients or families. I knew that the work the lab did was important, but I was no longer directly involved.

I went to nursing school for two semesters while I was also working as a secretary in a critical care unit. Life interfered, as it often does, so I did not complete nursing school either of the times that I attended. I continued to work in the hospital environment for 25 years in several capacities, such as EKG techs, cardiac monitor techs, and unit coordinators. I loved working in the hospitals. I was able to work hours that allowed me to be a mom to my two children, Shane and Nikky.

After my kids graduated from high school (and left me!!), I wanted a change in environment and career. I considered California and Florida and Florida won. I decided that I wanted to be directly involved in helping people feel better through touch. After some research into several schools, I went to Cortiva Institute of Massage Therapy. I chose Cortiva because they focused more on treating the person's healing and not just the steps of performing a massage. I learned to use my hands to effectively influence the way a person FEELS. I learned that touch could vary in pressure and pace to affect the muscle tissue in different ways. I learned neuromuscular therapy, myofascial release, hot stone massage, and sports massage. Upon graduation, I worked in a conservative chiropractic office for about a year. He really valued the beneficial effects that massage therapy has on soft tissue. It made his adjustments easier and longer lasting. It was eye opening into the fact that each person's body tells a different life story and that their needs were as unique as they are.

I joined the Florida State Massage Therapy Association so that I could be involved and to learn more about other ideas and modalities. I also wanted to network with other therapists in the event that a client may benefit from a different modality. Another benefit was that I may also fit the needs of their clients as well. Also, hanging out with other massage therapists is always interesting.

While working at the chiropractic office, I fell in love with my husband. We went to massage therapy school at the same time, but didn't interact with each other. He owned a massage practice in St. Petersburg called, The Peaceful Warrior Massage. We shared many of the same ideas and philosophies of touch therapy and helping others. I wanted to be a part of that environment, not to mention that I'd get to spend more time with him and be closer to home. I joined him and learned some new skills...more like I learned a total new way of life!!! I now understand things, such as payroll, taxes, scheduling, hiring, marketing, and creating a unique business profile that appeals to our clients. I think it's important here to note that many of these things I learned through trial and error, while others I learned through various groups that I joined. I became a member of the St Petersburg Chamber of Commerce. They offer many classes to their members to help build and grow a small business. I also participated and graduated from the Entrepreneurial Academy, a 10-week, intensive, small business course. I hired a business coach, Barry Foster, who helped me learn to manage my time more effectively and to delegate the tasks that I didn't want to do, or that someone may be more skilled at doing.

I now feel that I am able to help others both directly and indirectly. As a massage therapist, I provide the direct care through my touch and interaction with each of my clients. As a business owner, I am able to help others indirectly through the work of the other therapists here. I provide a job opportunity to those that want to fit into this approach to therapy.

I talk to all my clients and they talk to me and ask me lots of questions. I don't know the answers to most, but I love to find the answers! I have a network of other professionals that I can consult with both within this office and outside of it. I often will research more information about a specific issue or beneficial practices for my clients.

After five years of regularly sending my clients out to other offices for other healthcare services, we decided to expand into a wellness center by bringing in other practitioners in to our office. We have a doctor of Oriental medicine who offers acupuncture and herbal remedies, as well as tui na. We have a fitness trainer on staff as well that can suggest corrective exercises to help improve posture. We offer reflexology and SMRT (Spontaneous Muscle Release Therapy).

I have continued my education in therapy as well and now offer Himalayan salt stone massage and MediCupping. Salt is an amazing mineral that sometimes has an even more amazing effect in massage by restoring vital trace minerals and balancing the electromagnetic field. This protocoled massage is as calming to the mind as it is to the body. MediCupping is also called vacuum therapy. Using a machine to create suction through a hose, the cups pull the soft tissue away from the bone. It really opens up the pathways for blood flow and the nerves to function optimally. I find that I am really able to personalize each session because I have a lot of tools (massage modalities) in my tool box.

One of our therapists is the massage therapist for the Tampa Bay Rowdies, our local, professional soccer team. He is really involved in helping the players stay healthy and recover from any injuries they may incur while practicing and playing their games.

Somewhere along the way, I met Deserie Valloreo, founder of the Holistic Network of Florida. And no, this is not an attempt to brown nose or anything. I took a class on how to communicate with plants. I had no idea what to expect. All of the classes I had ever taken were through a huge hospital or college. This was nothing like that. She spoke from the heart and you could tell she didn't have a scripted speech that a committee had told her what she could and couldn't say. Deserie talked to each of us about how we felt. She inspired me and helped me realize that I could follow my own path in the holistic approach. I joined her network of other holistic practitioners. In the past, I have worked in the more traditional health environments, such as hospitals and clinics. When I could directly interact with the patients, I really felt like I could make a positive difference. But, I also felt restricted by the lack of time that I could spend with each one. The more traditional medical treatment plans of medicine and surgery in hospitals didn't always result in the patient FEELING better.

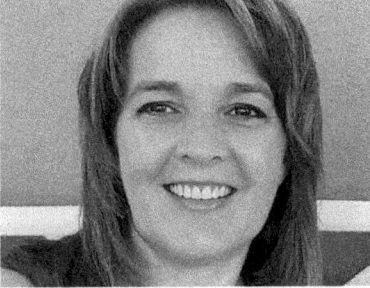

I choose to work in the field of massage therapy and holistic approach because I feel that it gives the client more, and often better choices to feel better. Most conditions are preventable through holistic approaches; most are also treatable this way. I really feel like I am able to offer the best prevention and treatment to a wide variety of common problems through the work that we provide in our office.

Lena Roberts, LMT, NMT
Peaceful Warriors Wellness Center, LLC
19 Dr. MLK Jr Street South
St Petersburg, FL 33705
727-822-8866
www.peacefulwarriorswellness.com

CHAPTER 11

FROM A MOTHER'S HEART:
UNEXPECTED CALLING

by Deborah R. Hutchinson, Functional Nutritionist, MS, BS, CHHC

"I am thankful for my struggle because without it, I wouldn't know my strength." - *Unknown*

Our tides had been turned. It was on a Wednesday in October, the year was 2005 when we received news our sons, along with several other kids had ingested a poisonous plant. Death knocked on my oldest son's door that evening, but by the grace of God, he survived. It wasn't until the next evening sitting in his hospital room when an outbreak occurred in the next room. The teenager who had been hallucinating for over 24 hours had broken the straps that secured him safely to his bed. It was complete chaos! Just moments before, two nurses from the ER were telling me they, along with several hospital staff the night before, were praying for my son, as they described, his heart was on the verge of exploding. That moment was intense for me to hear as a mom. After the dust settled in the next room, I sat back in my chair contemplating the recent events. I bravely asked, "Lord, I know you did not just allow my (our) world to be turned upside down for nothing. What do you need me to do?" I opened my bible and it fell on a scripture I wasn't familiar with: "You intended to harm me, but

God intended it for good to accomplish what is now being done, *the saving of many lives*. So then, don't be afraid, I will provide for you and your children…"(*Genesis 50:20-21, niv*). In the midst of these two verses lay my answer, "*the saving of many lives!*" It wasn't about us after all, but somehow I knew in that moment of my life, none of our lives would ever be the same. But, regardless of what we were about to walk through, we were all going to be OK.

It wasn't until nine months later sitting in an emergency room 14 hours from home while on vacation in Disney, that I knew my tides had turned indefinitely. This time, it was my youngest son whose mental/emotional ability was being seriously compromised. I didn't even know it was possible. There were many moments I had to remind myself to breathe. The boundaries that appeared to be broken in the spiritual realm were beyond my comprehension. My brain could not fully grasp what was happening. Just 24 hours before he went missing, it was almost midnight! We discussed the possible route to take to find him, but then I said, "Wait! God knows exactly where he is. I'm asking him!" Within five minutes, the front desk called and said, "There is a police officer here to take you to your son." We ran as fast as we could to the front of the resort. The police officer said, "Only one of you can go." As I got out of the car and began to walk closer, I stopped! I had to compose my thoughts and remind myself of a scripture. "Be still and know that I am God!" (*Psalm 46:10, niv*). As I drew closer, this person sitting on the back edge of an ambulance was not my son. I had never heard anything like this before. We gathered him up and took him back to the resort. We drove him to the hospital emergency room the police officer suggested. "It is further away, but probably not as busy," she said.

As we entered the emergency room to the receptionist desk, I looked up and read the sweetest words. It said, "As Jesus takes care of you, so do we." During our time in the emergency room, I sought answers once again. This time I said, "Lord, I don't know how to help my son. Please give me wisdom to know how to help and endure this with him." I pulled my bible from my purse. The Lord provided me three instructions that I still continue to abide to this day: "Rejoice in HOPE, be patient in tribulation, and be constant in prayer." (*Romans 12:12, esv*). In these early moments, I knew it was going to take more than my human ability as these events unfolded before my eyes. Over the years, I have kept these three instructions close to my heart, I've posted them all over my mind so that I would not enter one day without knowing there was something tangible I could do.

I've never known pure satisfaction until the Lord set me in the direction of my true life purpose: to provide HOPE and his healing to those who are often ostracized because of an addiction and/or mental/emotional struggle. I never knew the depths of pain until I witnessed my own son and others experiences, but they have been my source of motivation to move me forward into this unexpected calling. I struggled to find the words for the pain. I asked the Lord to help me define this pain. He spoke to my heart, "My child, this pain cannot be found in the heart. It is as if a sword went through, by-passed the heart, and pierced to the inner depths of your very soul. It is ingrained in the memory of your soul! I placed it there so your passion to help others would allow you to see through spiritual eyes and be able to experience the depths of their pain. Because it is only through these experiences that you can truly understand the depths of another's pain." The scripture to solidify his words is found in Luke 2:35, "…And a sword will pierce your own soul too." These words were said to Mary when Jesus was still a baby, but would play out 33 years later as Mary stood at the foot of the cross of her beloved son. So, just like Mary's pain on the day of redemption, the pain in a mother's heart for her child, every child, regardless of age would be felt to the same degree of intensity every time a child suffers the pains of this world. This pain can mobilize us into action or it can cripple us to utter despair. The choice is yours. I choose action.

Little did I know what lay ahead, but one thing for sure, I knew it was going to be OK! Out of desperation, I threw myself into researching every possible solution I could find. I was determined to find an answer! I knew to the inner most depths of my soul there had to be another way. I would not give up until I had answers for him. About seven months into this nightmare, I found The Pfeiffer Treatment Center, founded by Dr. Carl C. Pfeiffer, a maverick in the field of mental health and nutrition. We made the 16-hour trip to embark on our first introduction to an orthomolecular approach. After several functional medicine lab tests; from heavy metal toxicity to pyroluria disorder, we headed back home. I took the lab test to every single appointment. I knew what I had in my hands with this test held a critical piece of the puzzle, but NO ONE paid any attention. NO ONE would listen to his (our) story. NO ONE!!! I was told point blank, he would always have to take the medications for the rest of his life and to begin looking into state hospitals. I refused to believe my perfectly healthy son would never get well. He would overcome this horrific experience! He would be healthy again! And if they were not going to help him, I would. This led me to close my mortgage company and go back to school to embark on an educational journey leading me to obtain a doctorate in a clinical nutrition-centered functional medicine approach. I didn't know how or what it all looked like in the beginning, so just like everything else I've done in life, I threw myself out in to what seemed to be an ocean and began to swim in a wholistic direction. I've heard many times in life your true calling is the thing you've encountered frequently. The passion burns so deep inside of you that not only can you not let it go, but it won't let you go either.

Several years before, our kids wanted to create a surfing product line, hence the name of my company, Turning Tides, LLC. I said, "This is a great idea, but *we need to be different.*" Little did I know this conversation several years before would be the catalyst to us not just owning a surf product line, but one where we would offer support and HOPE to those who struggle with life challenges; all stemming from our family's own journey through pure hell.

I quickly realized changing a seriously broken system may not be the route to take, but instead I lean more towards a quote by Buckminster Fuller, "You never change things by fighting the existing reality. To change something, build a new model that makes the existing model obsolete."

In the process of attempting to find healing for our loved one through modern psychiatry, we only found more chaos and turmoil in every direction we turned. A functional medicine model offered us a whole new world of possibilities. Where modern psychiatry offered us doom and gloom with a possibility of no hope, the functional medicine route offered us HOPE in the healing of the whole person: Spirit - Soul - Body!!!

We are all prisoners to something but for many, being a prisoner to a drug that controls their mind is a reality. For others, it is their own brains that have been hijacked and kept them locked in a cage, and for others, perhaps it's a diagnosis to an autoimmune disorder that has them entangled in heavy chains of despair. Regardless of the prison, a functional medicine approach potentially has the key to unlock the suffering. We do not believe there is only one solution, but many probable solutions. It would seem the possibilities are limitless in some aspects. However, the one thing I've learned to be critically important is to address each client with a bio-chemical individuality concept in mind. God made every single one of us unique. We are not just a set of organs individually separated. Instead, we are a finely-tuned orchestra, where precision of incorporating all body systems together to bring harmony into place is a profound and accurate concept when it comes to restoring one's health.

In addictions, neurobiological and autoimmune disorders, there are often a lot of missing and broken pieces, such as the broken gut-brain connection, missing micronutrients, which are needed for biochemical pathways to function optimally, and epigenetic factors, such as environmental, lifestyle, and nutritional factors. The heart-brain connection is relevant, as is potential genetic factors. Your story is relevant!!! All of these areas are foundational to both physical and mental health. Lifestyle changes need to occur, such as providing tools and support for coping with stressful events, relaxation, breathing, meditation, prayer, physical activity, and more. A functional medicine practitioner's tool kit goes way beyond nutrition, but reaches into locating the root cause as to why you have the diagnosis in the first place. We acknowledge the innate way our body and brain were originally designed and how it is structured to function as a whole. Our comprehensive approach can help you reduce and/or eliminate stress, sleep disturbances, pain, brain fog, weight, fatigue, hormonal imbalances, emotional and addictive behaviors, and so much more. Every area of our lives can inhibit recovery and the healing process. Our hope is for our clients to be able to reduce and/or eliminate the need for a Band-Aid approach that only attempts to cover up a festering wound. But instead, utilize the power of God's "farmacy," made up of real, whole foods to include micronutrients, herbs, and things like essential oils.

Being facilitators of change, we utilize information based in nutrigenomics, epigenetics, methylation factors, and genetics to create a comprehensive plan of action for the individual. There is a reason for physical and/or mental/emotional struggles. The good news is, there is now a viable solution to locate potential root causes through a functional medicine approach.

Isaiah 66:13 "As a mother comforts her child, so I will comfort you..."

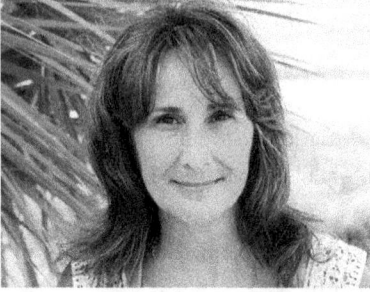

Debbie holds a master's degree as a Functional Medicine Clinical Nutritionist and is currently in the process of obtaining a doctorate in Clinical Nutrition. Her interest is in providing viable, evidence-based, natural alternative solutions to those who struggle with addictions, neurobiological and autoimmune disorders. Her specialized training is centered heavily in bio-chemistry, chemistry, and the intricate details of how the body and brain function optimally when it is provided the right nutritional and lifestyle support. She loves being able to provide her services through a tele-wellness platform, which allows her to help support clients, regardless of their geographical location.

Deborah R. Hutchinson Functional Nutritionist M.S., B.S., CHHC
Turning Tides, LLC
Debbie@turningtides.us
843-864-5018
www.turningtides.us
www.facebook.com/Turning-Tides-Surf-515830068517389/

CHAPTER 12

ADDICTION RECOVERY - TRANSFORMING DARKNESS TO LIGHT

by Jamey Kowalski, E-RYT200

It was May of 2011.

The time was about 1:00 p.m. and the room was too bright, even with the blinds closed. The air was heavy. I didn't smell good and for hours had been fighting to go back to sleep. I wanted to get up but simply could not. When I woke again, I turned over onto my other side and curled up into the fetal position, crying uncontrollably.

I was completely, utterly alone. My relationship of twelve years was gone; not my choice. Over time, I had pushed away family and then even close friends. I felt paralyzed and helpless. At that moment of desperate isolation, as I struggled to breathe between fits of sobbing and shaking, I wanted just two things: more alcohol to feel better, and to never drink again.

This was the real me. Not the outside me, the one I projected to the world. The one that said, "I'm OK" when someone asked how I was doing. This was the me that was drowning in fear, who had abandoned all parts of himself at the deepest level. The feeling of disconnection couldn't even be described, except to say, this was my rock bottom.

Other alcoholics and addicts have had far worse bottoms, suffering consequences way beyond what I did. But in recovery I've learned that each story is different, and that it takes what it takes for each of us to discover the "gift of desperation." And to find the truth which so many before us have found… that in the depths of this darkness and despair lies the seed of healing and renewal, of the transformation possible in life.

I'm forever grateful to have connected with an amazing counselor who helped me understand that I wasn't fundamentally flawed and broken. In fact, she helped me see that the alcohol served as self-medication, which may very well have prevented much more destructive forms of self-harm. It worked to soothe my pain, until it didn't anymore.

The community of Alcoholics Anonymous, although it doesn't resonate with everybody, offered me great respite and hope. These people really understood how a smart and energetic person could fall into the despair of addiction, despite having a lot of will power and success in other areas of life, such as work. I attended a lot of meetings and connected with a powerful web of support that kept me accountable and taught me that I was not alone in the struggle.

A bike crash leaving me with a broken collar bone four months into sobriety was a big challenge, yet I was able to persevere and by nine months was very active both riding and in the gym. As I began to lose the extra fifty pounds accumulated during years of alcohol abuse and related inactivity, my mental energy began to return, along with physical health. Some light came back into my life and I realized it would probably be a good idea to balance some of the intense exercise with gentle stretching.

That's when I discovered yoga. I had taken a class here and there before, yet this time was different. I started to understand the practice on multiple levels beyond the good it was doing for my body and got a glimpse into how it might not only help me stay sober, but actually thrive for the rest of my life.

I began to realize how much overlap existed between this ancient discipline and relatively modern ideas about recovery from alcohol and drug addiction. For instance, at a morning AA meeting, I'd hear one of the wise old-timers with decades of sobriety share about what it really means to take it one day at a time, sometimes even moment-to-moment when cravings and urges arose. And then in the evening, I'd hear my yoga instructor guide us to truly dwell in a posture, focusing attention on the sensation of what was happening in the body, simply "one breath at a time."

Or, I'd hear my gifted yoga teachers speak about "edge." This is the place of balance where engaging a healthy challenge doesn't become self-bullying; the line beyond which we're actually doing harm to ourselves with the practice, both physically and mentally. Similarly, I'd hear in the AA meetings and from my counselor about not being too hard on myself; how the need to over-achieve and the intense pursuit of perfection in all areas of life could actually derail my recovery.

It's often said that when someone comes into recovery from addiction, there's only one thing that really needs to change... and that's everything. It became increasingly clear that yoga was not an old religion but a life philosophy of guidance, a universal framework of ideas and tools that are highly applicable in our world today. Yoga offered the keys to fundamental change and healing on all levels: mental, emotional, physical, and spiritual. I was learning what it really meant to have balance, the kind that goes way beyond standing on one leg.

Some of my previous ideas about balance obviously needed a lot of help. Over the course of 15 years, beginning before my drinking career really took off, I spent a lot of time studying nutrition. Moving this theory into practice, I discovered ways to easily integrate healthy eating and supplementation into a busy life. There were times, especially at the end, where my food choices were totally off the rails but by and large, I maintained pretty good patterns. Yet, what seemed balanced at the peak of my addiction doesn't look so sensible today. For example, knowing that alcohol was hard on the liver and that lemon juice was cleansing and detoxifying for it, I thought vodka with nothing but a ton of organic lemon juice and ice made from filtered water was a perfectly reasonable idea!

This was the real bear of addiction. What seemed logical and even justifiable, at least on the surface, was at the root, horribly rotten and disconnected. So as I learned about how yoga meant "connection," a long-term path of recovery from the darkness seemed more possible each day.

Honestly, I was afraid of relapse. Over the many years of my drinking, there were weeks, months, and even some years that I was able to stop. Yet, it never lasted. There was always some trigger, some situation or seemingly good reason to have "just a little." Inevitably, that small lapse of judgment would cascade until my drinking was again completely out of control.

In 2008, I graduated from an intense, two-year program in applied clinical herbal medicine with a special focus on the traditional Chinese system of diagnostics and formulation. The teacher, an acupuncturist, was very gifted and opened my eyes to the energy of interplay between mental and emotional health and how it showed up in the body. It was amazing to help nurture transformation for so many clients in the school's student clinic. Yet, even in feeling a call to the healing profession and gathering more skills toward its service, I was so far from my own healthy path that the inauthenticity was ripping me apart. It was a deeply incongruent dishonesty; a spiritual disconnect.

The practice of yoga and meditation became an ongoing exploration of the truth behind my behaviors and helped to repair that disconnect. It was simple, although not easy, to breathe fully and notice what was actually happening with the experience of being me, using "beginner's mind" to move away from judgment, expectation, and prediction. I learned to come back to the present moment and focus on the breath when my mind wandered off to the past or the future, which seemed to happen constantly. It was difficult work but became an essential part of keeping my life aimed in the direction of continued recovery from addiction.

Yoga's physical effect also revealed what is meant by the phrase, "the issues are in the tissues." Sometimes, tears would show up in certain postures when stored memories and related emotions began to flow, while other times there would be tremendous feelings of joy and serenity. As my body began to soften and open up more, so too did other aspects of my being. Darkness was giving way to light.

It was clear this powerful healing method could help a lot of people in my community, so I went to school to become a yoga instructor and now hold advanced certification earned by teaching over a thousand hours. I learned how to help many different types of bodies effectively leverage the practice for their highest good, and saw how a dramatic shift in health on many levels could occur for others, as it had for me.

The growth and popularity of online yoga classes through video lit the light bulb above my head. How many people recovering from addiction could be reached and helped if I shared my knowledge online? Yet this required more continued work on the regret, guilt, and even shame about my past in order to be OK with putting myself out there to the entire world as a recovering alcoholic.

However, all my areas of expertise, including a background in technology work aligned to point in this direction. Through many conversations over the years with my peers in recovery, I'd learned there is a real desire for understandable information about complementary, holistic health tools. Even more importantly, there is a need for guidance in how to use them in a way that leads to balance, rather than overwhelm. It was clear this work was mine to do, regardless of the obstacles.

Countless people can be helped with everyday tools for addiction recovery, especially if the knowledge is presented online in a way that can be applied simply, one day at a time, in order to create positive, lifelong habits. I teach how to move beyond the darkness of addiction and transform by growing balance in recovery using yoga, qigong, meditation, mindfulness, nutrition with practical food choices, and appropriate herbal medicine.

I've known many people who are now in the ground because of addiction and relapse. Maybe you also know someone whose life has been impacted by the problem. Sometimes I recall the feeling of that day in bed when, although I didn't really want to die, I had absolutely no idea how to live. I'm grateful to have been shown the path of transformation, and to have both the skills and opportunity to help others who are suffering discover a solution for themselves.

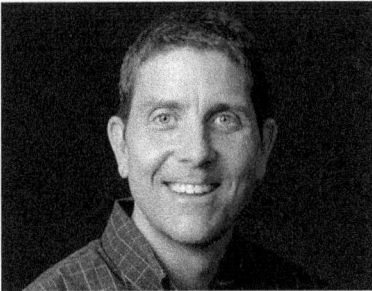

Jamey Kowalski is a recovering alcoholic helping people in all types of addiction recovery to get and keep their lives together using holistic health tools. He teaches yoga, qigong, meditation, mindfulness, nutrition with practical food choices, and appropriate herbal medicine. These everyday solutions enabled him to move beyond a dark time, grow balance in life, and remain free from alcohol since 2011. He's extremely grateful for the benefits of ongoing sobriety, including improved health on all levels: mental, emotional, physical, spiritual, and social. Jamey is very passionate about his calling to assist others along this path of transformation.

Jamey Kowalski, E-RYT200
www.GrowingBalance.com
www.facebook.com/GrowingBalance
Jamey@GrowingBalance.com

CHAPTER 13

HOLISTIC APPROACH TO HORMONE REJUVENATION: WHY THE CAUSE AND SOLUTION FOR HORMONE IMBALANCE IS ALL AROUND US

by Paige Clarke, CNHP, CA

I would guess I am not alone when I say my arrival at a "holistic lifestyle" was inspired by a personal challenge. Indeed, from what I have observed many of us in this field arrive here because we struggle to fix ourselves and/or loved ones.

I have a family lineage of brilliant and caring medical professionals. College led me to a sales and marketing career in the healthcare field. Not long in to it, I realized what was being practiced was "sick-care" and "health-cost" containment; neither of which fostered health and well-being in my mind. Medical intervention in emergencies and acute situations made sense to me but in wellness, prevention, and chronic issues, I just wasn't buying what they were selling. I trusted my intuition, grandma's remedies, and the adage, "a pinch of prevention is worth a pound of cure" at my very core. Thankfully, I had enjoyed excellent health and resilience, until the one event that stands in my mind and was a catalyst in the shift in my health and career.

I became ill after a long flight, preceded in hindsight by an extended period of burning the candles at both ends. After a few days of not successfully throwing it off as I usually did, I went to the doctor's office. The diagnosis was walking pneumonia and pleurisy and I was given antibiotics and codeine to calm the cough and ease the pain. After a week or so, I was back to work but my energy still waned. It didn't return as expected and in fact, in a few weeks I began to feel continual lethargy, body aches, and crushing tendonitis in my elbows. I simply could not get out of bed. When I did, I felt as if I had been hit by a huge truck. To add insult to injury, I was also perimenopausal and these symptoms combined were really delivering a double whammy.

I couldn't help but notice that I had never had muscle pain and fatigue like this before this incident and my visit to the doctor. At a follow up checkup, I questioned my doctor about the medications he had prescribed and he dismissed the idea that they would be contributing to my symptoms. I am curious and love connecting dots. I decided to do some research and I was quite disturbed by what I found. I was prescribed an antibiotic called Levaquin. When I explored the safety data sheets for Levaquin, I learned it is in a class of drugs, along with Cipro, called Fluoroquinolones. This class of drugs has documented side effects and even black box warnings. Please learn more about this dangerous class of antibiotic and protect yourself and your family. In short, it is a fluoride-based drug that depletes magnesium and leads to tissue damage, especially tendons, ligaments, and more. Magnesium is a crucial mineral in many functions in the body. Magnesium depletion also impacts the adrenal hormones and hormone balance in general. I began to see the downward spiral in my health spurred on at least in part by this dangerous drug. I somehow knew I needed to get back to trusting my intuition, grandma's remedies, and embrace nature-cure to re-cultivate my own wellness. It took a few months to really grasp the snowball effect that had happened in my body. In reality, it took me a few more years to recover from the fluoroquinolone damage. The stress from this incident and the hormone imbalance issues persisted, yet I was determined to find a solution.

It is apparent that what I have "unlearned" versus what I have "learned" has impacted me the most.

What does it really mean when we say we have a hormone imbalance or deficiency? After all, hormone "replacement" seems to be all the rage with anti-aging clinics on every corner. I really wanted to know why this was becoming such a big issue and such big business! How did we all become deficient? Why are these hormones not activating in our bodies? Shouldn't we be restoring function versus replacing function? Is there something that is creating interference, or are we not in the right environment to create them?

I had questions. I dove down the rabbit hole and began to really question the difference between hormone rejuvenation and hormone replacement. The truth I found is that there is really nothing natural about replacement, even with so called bio-identical hormone replacement therapy. These are in essence drug therapy that are manufactured or compounded. The administration of these products long-term will interfere with our natural feedback loop and innate chronobiology. This brilliant, natural circadian rhythm system we have is actually driven by time and light, and is the best compounding pharmacy on earth. What happens when we replace instead of restore? Replacement is when we add things; imposters actually, to supposedly help our body do what it is supposed to do. However, using these synthesized bio-identical compounds just does not work as planned. The static exogenous dosage interferes with the natural feedback loop, delivering the message that there is plenty of the substance in the body. This build up or toxicity, ironically, is in fact, the opposite of anti-aging. As a result of the imposter's presence, your own endogenous production of hormones is shut down or suppressed even further. Static replacement is true aging because we stop or own production as our glands involved in our built-in pharmacy literally go to sleep. Communication is disturbed in our cells and usually after a few months of replacement, the same or new symptoms appear. Even worse, there are too many things that can go wrong and one of them is cancer. Even though the Women's Health Initiative was utilizing equine-based synthetic hormones, it was proven that replacement created undesirable outcomes of cancer, gallstones, blood clots, and strokes. The results of mass bio-identical replacement are just not all in; their widespread use is becoming the study by default.

For me, I could see the inherent risks and problems replacement could cause in the body. I became intrigued with finding a more adaptive, holistic approach beyond hormone replacement, embracing true hormone rejuvenation. What exactly is rejuvenation? Hormone rejuvenation occurs when we eliminate the things that are interfering with our body being able to do what it was designed to do. Rejuvenation happens when we are making hormones on our own in the proper amount, and at the proper time. This is actually simple for the body, but we have created confusion due to an increasingly artificial, toxic world. The stress of our environment impacts the function of crucial organs and glands involved in the process of hormone production.

You can't fix a problem in the same environment that created it.

So how did I begin a holistic hormone rejuvenation program? I believe our bodies are magnificent creations whose creator makes no errors! I personally decided Mother Nature knows best and I wanted her to run the show. So I engaged… with her.

I realized that I had become so busy that I had neglected to connect with nature as often as I had in the past. This had caused an imbalance in my natural clock. Nature achieves balance through the change of seasons. So it takes time. We need time to regain balance as well. After a few months, my approach resulted in my hormones coming into a normal range and balance. I began to feel like myself again. My method could be called a quantum approach. This means the result of doing many small things creates an even greater overall result. To further clarify, just a few "extra" ordinary things can produce "extraordinary" results.

Why did I say the cause and remedy for hormone imbalance is all around us? Because it is; it is our environment. We need more of the good stuff and less of the bad stuff to achieve balance. We have to add more authentic nature interaction and eliminate engaging in the non-native aspects of our environment.

Do you:
- Walk barefoot to absorb earth's magnetism?
- Allow the Sun to dance on your skin and in your eyes each sunrise and sunset?
- Rehydrate your trillions of cells with good water so the Sun can do its magic inside?

Do you avoid:
- Being in artificial hormone disruptive blue lighting after sunset?
- Non-native EMF sources (Wi-Fi and cellphones) as much as possible, especially while sleeping?

I found that the answer is not found in a pill but all around us in how and when we interact with our environment. Go *outside* to be healthy *inside*!

When we realize the impact of our environment on our health, we learn that to enjoy big quantum results, we must look to change the little things:

How and *when* do you eat, drink, move, sleep and think?

What I did differently to recover and now share with others in my rejuvenation programs is that it matters when you do these simple things, not just how you do them. For example, this is fascinating: we create a great deal of our sex hormones in the early morning sunrise hours if we allow the sunlight to safely hit our eyes. It is also the time nature synthesizes melatonin via this light in our eyes for better sleep at night. Conversely, staring at the bright-as-day blue light of the TV into the late night hours disrupts the release of this melatonin, resulting in less than optimal sleep. Less sleep results in less rejuvenation and repair. Nature has her clock and when we synch with her, things flow better.

You too can facilitate hormone rejuvenation by getting in touch with your chronobiology and the circadian rhythm of Mother Nature. I created a method that helped me stimulate my "in-house" compound pharmacy for a safe effective "holistic approach" to hormone rejuvenation. The cause of hormone imbalance is the environment; the solution is also found in the environment. Beautifully simple isn't it? Restore, don't replace by reconnecting with the environment all around you. This is the crucial step in the true art and science of anti-aging.

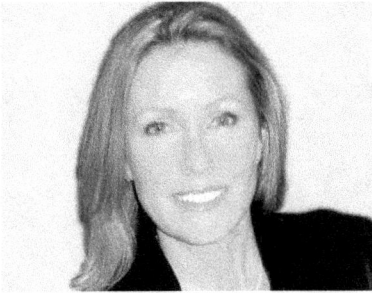

I'm a passionate advocate for healthy living and self-healing empowerment. My mission is to enlighten and empower you to ignite your unique healing power within. I have an insatiable appetite for knowledge. With over thirty certifications and counting, I would love to share the wisdom and secrets I have learned with you.

In my work with people, I combine ancient wisdom with modern science. I specifically rely on the study of epigenetics, or "above the genes," which proves your genes do not control your destiny, you do! Thus, you are powerful and can defy your DNA! I will show you how to use food, nutrients, frequencies, essential oils, light, sound, movement, breath, water, and positive thoughts to naturally heal your body and mind. So if you're ready to take charge of your destiny, let me guide you on your own personal healing journey toward limitless health.

For my coaching clients, I offer specific rejuvenation programs and consultations via phone, Skype, or in person at my office in delightful downtown Dunedin, Florida. Connect with me at www.PaigeClarke.com.

CHAPTER 14

THE QUEST FOR THE MIND-BODY CONNECTION

by Gina Carrillo, Mind-Body Medicine Practitioner

According the American Medical Association (AMA), approximately 80% of health issues are stress related and WebMD reports that 75-90% of doctor's visits are for stress-related ailments. But yet, according to the American Psychological Association (APA), only 1 in 5 or about 20% of us use activities designed to rid of us stress, or at least manage it.

What does this say about us as a society? We are ill, stressed out, and need help! I don't know about you, but I don't need statistics to prove to me how stressful life is and I have learned that stress has indeed been the cause of all of my health issues.

The good news is, we have the power to heal ourselves. This may sound like some cheesy kumbaya statement but I am living proof the power of the mind-body connection is powerful enough to create and heal pain and disorders. Our minds don't discriminate between reality and obsessing over something. So when we worry, our bodies think it's a real threat and respond accordingly. So, if we can cause the stress response merely by thinking about it, we also have the ability to harness the power of our minds and listen to the wisdom of our bodies to heal ourselves. I am by no means suggesting not seeing a doctor, but if you have chronic pain or health issues and you can't find a solution, it is my sincere hope my story inspires you to find the answers.

Without boring you with my entire life story, let me highlight some key areas to provide frame of reference for what's to follow.

Growing Up

I had a normal life I supposed you could say until I was about seven when my parents divorced. We went from a two-parent, traditional household with a nice house to a poor, single-parent small apartment in a not-so-nice part of town, and a mostly absent father. That is also when I started gaining weight and have never been able to have a normal weight since. My mother worked long hours to support us and we became "latchkey" kids. As I gained weight, others made fun of me and I retreated. I've only recently realized through lots of introspection and mind-body techniques how much these early years have played a role in my self-esteem, self-worth, and confidence, and the disorders that plagued me in my adult years.

Adulthood

As a young adult, I developed some intermittent digestive issues but didn't know anything about IBS back then and thought it was related to certain foods (e.g., eggs). Fortunately, it wasn't as bad as it would be later in life, so I mostly ignored it and kept going.

I put myself through college and before I graduated, became pregnant with my daughter. Her father left, so I raised her on my own, and after three years in a horrible job, I moved from Indiana to Florida to start a new job and a new life. I worked full-time and also did a lot of freelance writing, editing, and teaching on nights and week-ends; burning the candle on both ends trying to get ahead.

Around this same time, I developed knee problems (grinding and instability), osteoarthritis, and my digestive issues worsened. Conventional doctors couldn't help me with the digestive issues, so I saw a holistic doctor who told me about IBS and leaky gut. Unfortunately, there wasn't much even the holistic doctor to do for me then. My weight problems persisted as well. So, I took Motrin for the pain and swelling, Imodium for the gastrointestinal issues, dieted and exercised, and kept going. Over the course of the following 10 years or so, my knees worsened, requiring three surgeries in an attempt to prolong the need for total knee replacements. I was still working out (to my best ability) to try to lose weight but it took its toll on my knees. I lost more and more mobility, could no longer squat, lunge, climb stairs, stand, or walk for any length of time without a lot of swelling and pain. So, I took lots of Motrin (which wasn't good for my gut either) and kept going.

Do you see a pattern here?

Before the second surgery, I met the love of my life, and though the situation wasn't ideal with him in the Bahamas and me in Florida, I was happier than I had ever been. We would visit each other as often as we could but after a few years, it started to become a source of stress and discord. However, I was able to finally lose some weight but the IBS was ever present. So, I just kept taking the Imodium and kept going.

After my second knee surgery, I began physical therapy but soon after, I started experiencing extreme pain in my lower back, followed by my neck. I could barely move without extreme pain. And since my left knee was still recovering, my right side and knee took the brunt. I literally didn't have a good leg to stand on!

I was referred to a spinal specialist and after undergoing lots of X-rays, imaging, tests, and assessments, they found the following: spondylolisthesis, degenerated discs in my lower back, four herniated discs in my neck, spinal stenosis, slight curvature of the spine, and carpel tunnel. Their findings scared the hell out of me! They prescribed physical therapy, massage therapy, stimulation machines, additional tests, supplements, and pain medication. And just when I thought it couldn't get any worse, the IBS worsened, and I developed Fibromyalgia and tremors in my head and right hand, and had to see a neurologist.

After several months, my right knee was so bad, I had my third surgery just months after my left knee surgery. The pain was by far the worse out of all three surgeries and worse than all of my chronic pain combined. The recovery was long (a year) and excruciating. Every day became about managing pain and IBS, doing physical therapy, and seeing doctors and specialists. I feared never being "normal" again and grew depressed, exhausted from the pain, frustrated my now fiancée was in another country, and the only family I had around was my daughter. All of this added to the reservoir of stress, already at capacity.

When my fiancée next visited several months later, we decided to elope. This meant he could stay in the country but couldn't work until we went through immigration, a costly and lengthy process, and more stress. I was happy to finally have him with me, but the day before he arrived, my disabled mother also moved in. Soon after, I was promoted in my job and though it was a welcome promotion, it came with a huge amount of pressure and workload.

With all of these added responsibilities and pressures, I developed even more ailments, including rheumatoid arthritis, chronic yeast infections, even worse IBS, more weight gain along with hypothyroidism, and anxiety. I was struggling to stay afloat, had no outlets (I could no longer work out), and everything was building up inside.

Making the Connection

After almost an additional year, nothing the physical therapists or doctors did worked and my insurance would no longer approve the visits and care. Fortunately, my massage therapist told me about a book a friend of hers read to get rid of his back pain. I had forgotten what it was like to not be in pain and have a normal life. I had a friend tell me my sparkle was gone and for the first time, I understood what it was like to be in so much pain, you'd rather end it all than endure another day. I had to force myself out of bed every day. I wasn't living anymore. I was merely existing.

I immediately bought the book my massage therapist recommended, called *Healing Back Pain: The Mind Body Connection,* by Dr. John Sarno and read it over the course of a few weeks. After just a few days, I was in less pain and after two weeks, the Fibromyalgia was totally gone. It was a ray of sunshine I hadn't felt in almost two years!

If you've never heard of Dr. Sarno, he was a rehabilitation doctor that revolutionized the world of pain and the relationship between the mind and the body. He discovered pain and other ailments he categorized as TMS (Tension Myositis Syndrome) could be eliminated by teaching patients about the mind-body connection. TMS ailments are extensive, ranging from allergies, arthritis, pain, migraines, high blood pressure, plantar fasciitis, IBS, and neuropathy, to possibly even cancer. These ailments are caused by the emotional response to stress, trauma, anger, guilt, anxiety, etc. So, in other words, the root cause of these ailments is emotion, not physical abnormalities. That's not to say that physical abnormalities don't exist. But for someone like me, I was able to rid myself of Fibromyalgia and other ailments by reading Dr. Sarno's book and doing a lot of inner work to uncover the true root cause. Remember I mentioned the stressors going on and the scary diagnoses, surgeries, etc.? Those were the root causes. And by suppressing the symptoms with medication, I was imploding.

It's not always as simple as this. It took a lot of digging internally and combining what I learned from Dr. Sarno and seeking out training and education in mind-body medicine to get to the bottom of some of it. I believe we store stress and emotional pain in our very fibers, which gives a whole new meaning to muscle memory! And it has been my experience, the more traumatic the life experience, the worse the symptoms are, the deeper the buried emotions go, and the harder it is to get rid of. Fibromyalgia was much easier to get rid of than the IBS. But, your experiences may be differ. Our life experiences are different and so too will be the ailment and the root cause it's connected to.

So, after reading the book, I had such a revelation because if I could get rid of fibromyalgia by reading a book and doing some inner work, what else could I accomplish? I went on a mind-body connection quest and found the Center for Mind Body Medicine, quickly enrolled in their Mind-Body Medicine training, followed by the advanced training to become a mind-body medicine practitioner. I learned so much about the repercussions of the stress response and the physiology behind it, as well as scientifically-proven techniques to manage stress and the impact it has on our body and minds.

I had a renewed vision on what I wanted to do the remainder of my life. But at the time, I was still holding down a very stressful job and lots of responsibilities at home. So I returned to my regularly scheduled programming and endured more stress, and the resurfacing of pain and additional ailments: more digestive issues and severe anxiety and panic attacks accompanied by severe IBS. I later discovered these more recent ailments were connected to the pressures of my new position and deep emotional hurt and insecurities tied to my childhood. The IBS was never about food intolerances, a leaky gut, or anything related to my digestive system. It took a while to figure this out, but when I did, it all went away. I should mention here that whole and plant-based foods, quality sleep, and the mind-body connection create the foundation for health and well-being. You can't have one without the others and have well-balanced health.

So, think of buried emotions like weeds. Stress and repressed emotions cause imbalances, leading to disorders. Conventional medicine and even some functional/integrative medicine treat the symptoms with drugs, surgeries, therapy, supplements, food restrictions, etc. These forms of treatment are the equivalent to just mowing over the top of the weed in an attempt to remove the unsightly part of it. Until you pull the weed out by its roots, it won't go away. However, there are also times when you don't even know emotions are buried because there is no outward symptom until something in life triggers it. Then there are others that have root systems so large and vast, it takes a bit more time to uproot.

Using all of my own experiences, what I've learned from studying and reading Dr. Sarno's works, and the hands-on training I received from the Center for Mind Body Medicine, I've created my own approach to mind-body wellness and stress and pain management called the *Mind-Body Manifesto.*

No one should feel powerless and at the mercy of their emotional and physical pain, or go through life stressed out. Sometimes we need a little help uncovering the root causes behind our ailments and learning how to dig them out, and that's where I come in!

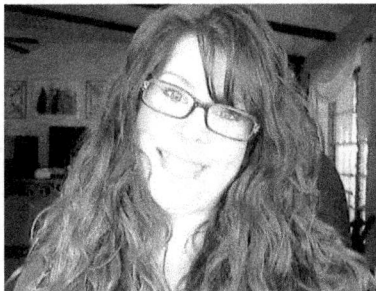

Gina has 24 years' experience in training, adult learning, project management, and instructional design, is a published author and editor, and has advanced training in mind-body wellness from the Center for Mind Body Medicine. Her background spans various industries including technology, healthcare, sales, finance, and more. Empowering others is Gina's passion. She offers educational talks for corporate and educational wellness events, group sessions, and individual coaching on how to leverage the mind-body connection using scientifically-proven techniques to help heal emotional and physical pain and illness, de-stress and relax, uncover and work through emotional blockages, and regain and maintain overall health and well-being.

Gina Carrillo, Mind-Body Wellness Practitioner
Mind-Body Manifesto
gina@wayseer.net
www.facebook.com/Mind-Body-Manifesto-1715390838766213/
www.linkedin.com/in/gina-carrillo-27a3896/

CHAPTER 15

CHANGE YOUR THOUGHTS TO HEAL YOUR LIFE

by Terri Cabral, Certified Life & Business Coach and
Spiritual Teacher

A few years ago, I went through some medical challenges that made me take a serious look at my life. I made good money and loved what I did, but as most of you have experienced in the past 10 years, corporate jobs were changing and not for the better. Profit was above caring and people become indispensable.

Being a sensitive person and seeing the way that people were being treated after they gave their all to make companies successful, made me literally sick. The stress was overwhelming and I collapsed to be put on bed rest by my doctor, my immune system had been compromised, and too many things were not looking good.

While on bed rest, I hired a life coach and started working at getting clarity about my future and the rest is history, when it came to my career.

I would like to share with you how I took control of my health. After seeing many doctors and not getting a lot of optimism or help, I decided to do a lot of research about alternative methods. I lived with my grandparents and aunts for some time as a child and they really believed in herbs and natural healing, so this felt very natural to me.

This was the start of my journey. Since there was no conventional healing for me and conventional practices made me feel like I should have no hope (for my own situation), I researched holistic modalities and doctors that would help; anything from eastern herbs, western supplements, health food stores, biofeedback, Reiki, natural oils, meditation, theta wellness, inspirational books, gratitude, prayer, and faith.

All the above methods helped, but one thing that I realized was that if I spoke about being sick and spent time with people that talked about me being sick, I would actually feel sicker. I also knew that when I went to the doctor, I came home feeling worse. Was there something connected to thinking, hearing, and speaking the words of sickness? I used to teach positive thinking to the people that I trained in the cosmetic industry. I knew this to a certain level and when things became very negative, people started to get sick, including me. I started looking into this at a deeper level. The correlation between thoughts, the words we speak, the emotions, and physiology. The medical community knows that an individual's state of mind has a lot to do with the healing process.

I read a lot about this subject, which is today one of my chosen inspirational talks to many groups. The mind is a sponge. Everything that we hear and believe stays stored in our subconscious mind. The more you hear it, the more you accept it. That is how we remember things and do certain things automatically, like robots. Have you ever driven home and don't really remember how you got there? You didn't pay much attention to it because this routine is already part of your programming.

Think of the mind like a computer's hard drive. Someone programmed those files. When you look for the information, it comes up fast. You don't need to do a lot of searching. It's there. Your mind works the same way. For instance, if you don't believe that you can make a living as an artist because you always heard that from your family or friends, you won't, unless you delete that file. Many artists make a lot of money because they have a different belief system. The information in the file might be, "I Am a successful artist. Everyone wants to own a piece of my art work." Do you see the difference? This is also called an affirmation. The words, "I Am" are extremely powerful. Therefore, what follows that should have power, presence, positivity.

This is how I started to change my thinking, feeling, and of course that changed my physiology, my health, and my outlook on life. I created paradigm shifts. I still have some challenges but I no longer dwell on them. I am not telling you to ignore your health, but I am telling you that you can change your thinking and feel better. The subconscious mind is like a garden. Thoughts and belief systems are planted there. According to the thought, you will either grow beautiful flowers or you will grow weeds. Flowers are prettier and give you a better feeling. The thought is the seed that creates feelings and emotions. Napoleon Hill said, "Whatever the mind of man can conceive and believe he can achieve." He wasn't talking about skill. He was simply talking about a belief system; the programming of our subconscious mind. Whether the thought is a higher frequency thought or lower, you will create it. So, we must be very aware of this moment because it will show up in your life.

We can look at times in our lives when we were in certain states of mind and remember what happened 90 days from then. Most likely it was a life experience of our belief systems.

During my difficult time, I started talking to myself. I know you are probably thinking that this is crazy, but it takes 100 positives to start to clear one negative. That's a lot of positives to put to work. Think of it as making deposits into your bank account and look at the negative thoughts as a withdraw from your bank account. If you keep up with too many of those, you will be bankrupt soon. Negative thoughts make the body and spirit feel drained. Mind, body, and spirit are all one.

My secret was this: if the thought was negative, I imagined a cancel or delete button to press and I would say, "delete, delete, delete" and replace it with a positive thought, such as, "I am healthy and strong." Tony Robbins says, "You must stand guard at the door of your mind." Therefore, I protected my mind, not only from myself but also from those who meant well, but were not helping. I did this all day. I replaced thoughts with affirmations (a phrase in present tense, as if it already happened). After a while, I would catch the full negative program before it came out and replace it immediately. I carried affirmations written on 3x5 cards according to what I thought needed to be changed and repeated them, often out loud. I posted them on mirrors, the refrigerator, etc. I was reprogramming my subconscious mind, not only for health, but also peace, happiness, and wealth.

Since I had to walk away from my income, I also had other concerns and fear (false evidence appearing real) sneaked in many times, along with the feelings of shame, not working a full-time job anymore, and the guilt of not bringing in the income. These three feelings are great companions. We were taught these emotions extremely well, depending on our upbringing and culture. People teach what they know. But our job now is to ask ourselves, does this feeling match my decision or who I am? Where is it coming from? When we get that awareness, then we must work at changing it. This was a tough one for me, but I must say, shame and guilt are no longer part of my life. That was my affirmation for years.

I learned that our thoughts and feelings have a frequency and that everything has vibration. Frequency emits waves (electromagnetic waves) like a radio does and attracts the same back to us, like a boomerang. What we put out, we get back. That is why the more I thought about being sick, the sicker I got. The frequency of this belief was attracting more of it. When you think happy thoughts, you feel happier because you lift the frequency and get more of that. The word, sick, is a lower frequency than the word, happy. Frequency charts can measure words. Change your thoughts, words, and feelings to heal your life.

I started to listen to my thoughts and my body. My body was talking to me all along but I was not listening. We have a natural GPS within us. All we need is already within us, but we don't always listen. So, when my body was saying enough, I learned that it was time to nurture my being (mind, body, and soul) and take time off to rest. This was not a common routine for me, since I always had things to do on my list, and for me at this time, this really meant doing absolutely nothing. In the past, I drove myself crazy, along with the people around me, my amazing family, husband, and sons. This was a precious life lesson.

I learned about the law of attraction and really put it to work. The right people started to show up in my life, I started manifesting things pretty quickly, and really believed that all my desired goals could come true. I am grateful to be able to say that many of my goals have come to fruition and also know that gratitude played a big part in it. I was happy to be grateful for many things, even when people on the outside couldn't see much of what I should be happy about. Prayer was a daily regimen with daily gratitude and journaling; it became a constant reminder of the good in my life. Everything that gave me joy that day, I wrote it down. This simple exercise made me more aware of my blessings. Our mind starts to absorb more of that and shows us more to be grateful for.

The true feeling of gratitude is the fastest way to move your life forward. Live in thankfulness and you will feel more joy. Think back on what brings you more joy and do more of that. It is OK to have more fun. This higher vibration will help you to be more creative, to be the authentic you that you were always meant to be, and enjoy life more. You are unique. There is no one like you. Only you can walk your path. That alone is a miracle.

Being a type A personality, I need to be a doer and accomplished. Times of solitude, especially meditation were not easy for me but these moments were my greatest teachers. The long to-do lists disappeared and I felt free, focusing more on what felt good and less on what didn't, released a lot of stress, and I acted with more trust and ease, and reacted less. My life took on more meaning. Everything started to fall into place because I changed my thoughts, changed my habits, believed, and trusted.

Without this transition in my life, I wouldn't be able to spend weekends with my family, I would not be flexible to go wherever we want to go, would not be at home every holiday, and getting my bachelor's and master's degrees would not have been a possibility. I also became a spiritual teacher, a Reiki master, an ordained minister, and chose to inspire others with my professional talks and coaching. My achievements were actually better and more meaningful and through my increased faith, I was guided to grow into the person that I am today.

Most of all, I am proud to be making a bigger difference, be more present, and help many people to live a healthier and more fulfilled life. I believe that we are all a spark of the Divine and that this greater power does not make mistakes. There was a bigger purpose for this change in my life and that was the only way for me to pay attention and make this shift. My detour was a gift from the Creator; one that I now take seriously to follow my life mission and leave my mark on this Earth.

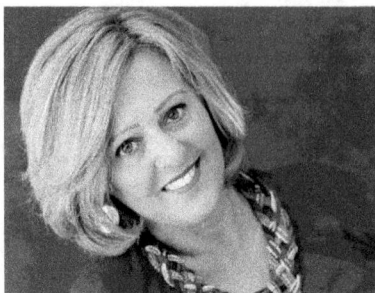

Terri Cabral is certified life and business coach, specializing in personal and business development, spiritual growth, and balance. She makes you aware of your belief systems and helps you create new paradigm shifts to shift your thinking and raise your frequency. She guides you to a greater success, a more fulfilling purpose-driven life, with real and practical steps. Through her coaching program, she helps you to awaken the giant within you; your authentic, more confident self that is ready to live a life of peace, joy, and success.

www.terricabral.com

terri@terricabral.com

www.facebook.com/terricaballifecoach

CHAPTER 16

SURVIVE AND THRIVE

by Saroeup (Sara) Im, Award-Winning Author, Speaker, and Holistic
Wellness Consultant

Have you ever experienced an abrupt change that would wreck your life?

I believe that life is not about what happens to us, rather it's about how we
handle it. Let me start by sharing a journey of my younger life and tell you
how I recovered from my near-death and painful experiences.

As a child growing up in Cambodia, I was secure, loved, and honored as the
first born of my parents. Once, Cambodia was a beautiful country with
beautiful, lush, tropical foliage with parrots, cranes, elephants, buffalos,
oxen, horses, bears, panthers, tigers, and deer. The people were peaceful
and tolerant. They loved their neighbors and enjoyed a community lifestyle.
The world knew Cambodia by the marvelous temple of Angkor Wat, one of
the seven wonders of the world; a breath-taking, huge stone monument
built over 1,000 years ago.

In April 1975, my beautiful tropical country experienced the most horrific
event in history. Then, I was 21 years old and my peaceful life turned upside
down abruptly without warning. I was attending college in the capital city of

Phnom Penh, while all of my family was hundreds of miles away. The Khmer Rouge Communists invaded Cambodia. They brutally imposed on the urban inhabitants an immediate evacuation from the centers of all cities. They shut down city life and every market place, restaurant, school, government office, and hospital, all lines of transportation, all lines of communication, and other aspects of civilized life. I was desperate and in a dire situation away from my family.

After walking in the heat for several weeks and being dishonorably relocated twice, I ended up in a rice field camp controlled by the armed Khmer Rouge soldiers. I endured four brutal years in a forced labor camp that became known as, "The Killing Fields."

One quarter of Cambodian population (over two million people) perished during the tyranny of the Khmer Rouge regime (1975- 1979).

As I got trapped in this camp, people were pushed to work unimaginable long hours in the rice fields under a scorching, hot sun from dawn all the way to night time. During that miserable time, we, the laborers received minimal food portions with no taste, nor nutritional value. Many of us in the camp became sick and I too became very sick. I had malaria, typhoid, swelling of my whole body, and then I became emaciated, like a skeleton covered with saggy rough skin. There was no medication to help me get better, no doctor, no clinic to help me recover. I was extremely weak. On top of that desperate situation, I became blind at night. This disorder was known in Cambodia as night blindness. I realized the lack of rest, lack of nutrition, and the lack of essential vitamins were the cause of damaging havoc to my body and my vision. I could not see anything at night, no matter how close I was to the light. When I became too sick to work, they moved me to a makeshift infirmary away from the working people.

When I arrived, I saw people there were very sick with more diseases than me. I had seen people in this makeshift infirmary die almost every day. I knew I would soon contract more diseases from others and I would die just like them. I realized I needed to get out of there to survive. I constantly thought about my family and I wanted to be with them. When I could not do anything to help myself get better, I began to search for a solution. Then, I remembered one of the stories my mom read to me before bedtime when I was very young. In this story, a mean person grabbed two children and a woman from another man and he dragged them and beat them up. God saw what happened and sent his angel to rescue the children and the woman from this mean man. From that story, I believed that God exists, and He is kind and compassionate. I have believed in God since then. At the time that I needed to survive, I prayed for God's help. I started to pray at night for God to help me stay alive and find my family. My body was too weak and too sick to survive, but my soul and my spirit were filled with my love for my family and my faith in God.

For a few weeks, I prayed. One day, I felt I had just enough strength to walk over to the other side where the working people stayed. When I got there, a work team leader saw me coming and she took me into her group. After observing me trying my hardest to keep up with the pace of work, she realized that I was very sick. Two days later, she found me a job in the kitchen. It was such a life-saver!!! I began to work in the kitchen. I got to have more food to eat, worked fewer hours, and worked in the shade instead of in the extreme heat. I soon began to feel better. I then realized that I had survived!!! I felt blessed that I had that chance to get out of the infirmary and was given a chance to work in the kitchen to overcome my deadly condition. After several months, when they saw me looking healthier, they dragged me out to work in the rice field again.

After four brutal years in this camp, I secretly asked a few god sisters in the camp to take a huge risk with me to escape from this ordeal. Thank God, we succeeded. We walked and found our way to my hometown. I tracked down my family and finally was reunited with them. My mother was in shock when she first saw me. To her, I looked like a walking skeleton. Nevertheless, she hugged me so tight and cried out, "My darling!!! I am so happy to see you alive!!!" The next day, my dad said, "I have been looking for you all these years. We thought that you were dead. We gave away all your clothes." Mom made all the good foods to remedy my shaggy frame. In only a few months of being pampered with the love of my family, time to rest, enough time to sleep and enough nutritious, organic foods, I recovered my health and shed off my numerous diseases. I believed my healing was the result of good nutrition, no more stress of dealing with harsh working conditions, no more exhaustion from unbelievable long hours under the brutal hot sun, and no more worrying about what happened to my loved ones. I am now grateful that I have fully recovered from that dark experience.

After one year in a happy reunion with my family, I was compelled to escape Cambodia to find safety in another country. Once again, God was with me; my escape was successful. After staying in the refugee camp for one year, I arrived in US in 1981. I received incredible support from the Christian community belonging to a few churches in Connecticut. I started my new life, learned the language, got a paying job, and started college.

Just before I graduated from college in 1987, I found myself in extreme stress and incredible emotional pain. My mom, my three brothers, my sister-in-law, and two toddler nieces escaped to Thailand. They arrived in a closed refugee camp. They were in hiding as illegal residents of the camp. My family was in a great danger. I began to seriously search for ways to ease my emotional turmoil. That was the time when my pastor's wife took the time to teach me the Bible precepts and one day, she showed me the Bible verse, John 3:16 "For God so loves the world that He gave his only son to die for us, whoever believe in Him will never perish but have an eternal life." When I saw and heard that, I thought to myself, *Wow, He gave His Life!!! He gave his ultimate possession! What else could I ask from Him?* I did not wait another minute. I accepted Jesus to be my Lord and Savior. As I continue my walk with Jesus and my search for healing, I found so many Bible verses that are so healing and comforting. I love Psalm 147:3 that reads, "He heals the broken-hearted and binds up their wound." That was me who was broken-hearted and suffered deep emotional pain.

Today, I am thankful that God has brought me so far. He saved me from my near-death illness, protected me during my dangerous escapes, and brought me to safety. He blessed me with wonderful, faithful Christian friends and churches to help me start my new life. And finally, I found the true joy to have Jesus in my life. I found peace in the Lord and I meditate on Bible verse, Psalm 30:2 "Oh Lord my God, I cried out to you, and you healed me."

I learned that our best state of health and happiness can be achieved from these basic factors:

We need love

When I struggled in the darkest days of my life in the rice camp, I remembered the love my family had for me. My deepest love for them gave me strength to keep on fighting to survive. We also find love in the community that we trust. When we focus on love, we can choose to forgive our enemies and let go of anger, bitterness, and resentment. Now that I know God better, I believe that God's unconditional love for us is priceless. Everyone can receive this love. It is so powerful!

We need hope

Hope is like the light in the darkness. My feeling of strong love gave me hope that I would make it through the toughest times. I had hope that one day, I would overcome my adversity. Without hope, you would not have motivation to achieve better goals in life. Hope is like gas for your car; without it, you cannot move forward. When we have hope, we have a positive perspective in life, and a positive perspective on life strengthens our hope.

We need physical health

The quality of our physical health determines the quality of our life. Everyone should fulfill his/her basic physical needs. These basic needs include quality food, proper, balanced nutrition, clean water, proper housing, adequate rest, enough sleep, less stress, and less toxics chemicals. Lately, I have observed that so many people don't eat good food anymore. They eat preserved canned food and packaged processed food or fast food. That means that you may fill your stomach, but there are little nutrients. We become too busy to prepare fresh meals for the family. We become too busy to have time for rest and sleep. We put ourselves in so much debt, we stress ourselves out to the limit to keep up with all the bills. We become too naive to think that big manufacturers would not compromise the health and safety of the consumers for their own greedy profits. They use harmful, toxic chemicals in personal care and household products.

We should be mindful of these unhealthy habits and make some positive changes to enjoy our good health and live our happy life. It is better to focus on prevention.

We should strive for these three basic foundations: hope, love, and physical health. They make up our whole being, which is composed of spirit, soul, and body.

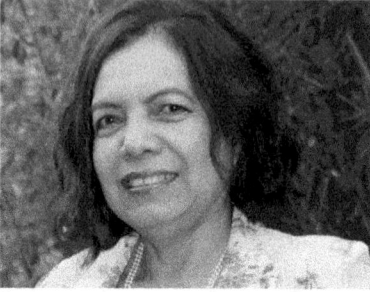

Thank you for reading my story to this point. My full survival story is described in my book, *How I Survived the Killing Fields, a Story of Hope, Love and Determination.* Along with my book, I speak to restore hope and change lives. You can reach me at www.saraim.com.

CHAPTER 17

AN INTEGRATED APPROACH: THE ROAD LESS TRAVELED

by Lisa Seward, Licensed Massage Therapist MA10898, Certified BodyTalk™ Practitioner

I want to inspire people to know there is a light at the end of the tunnel. Trauma may not stop you in life, unless you want to go that way, and forfeit your health and wellbeing. It might be a wakeup call to have you look at your life and be ready to get well. It is an inside job that can be motivated by your willingness to step up to the challenge. *Never give up* is my motto! I would hope to inspire you to challenge your body, your mind, and soul to want to get well! Do whatever it takes! It is possible to over-come all odds and see the other side of poor posture, pain, and to transform your old self to the new and improved model.

How do I know that it works? What makes me an expert in the field of trauma? I was born with a deformity, overweight, bullied for looking uniquely different, had cosmetic surgery, and a heart catheterization; all by the age of 12. Then, 25 years later, I was impacted by a four-car accident. I survived and now thrive. Trauma isn't any longer my friend, but just a reminder of years ago, where poor posture and rigidity held me prisoner - tight and less active in my journey to wholeness. My dream of good posture and being alive, taller, and straighter, were my claim to fame!

It was a wakeup call when I got rear-ended in 1994; twice within two months! I began seeing a chiropractor, who said after reading the X-rays, "You look like a 90-year-old!" *Really?* I thought to myself. I was only 37 years old! It was the first time ever that anyone really let me know how off my posture was! I thought, *It must have been the car accident!* Since I had worked for a chiropractor right after graduating from Tampa's Suncoast School of Massage Therapy in 1990, I never heard that comment in his office.

It happened on the way to do chair massage at the Safety Harbor Library's grand opening October 1, 1994. Then, two months later, I was rear-ended by a huge, white car coming right at me, as I saw her in the rear-view mirror. She was not slowing down as I waited for the light to change. The impact on my small Geo Prizm nearly totaled it, as it pushed me into the car ahead of me. The pattern continued until the first car was hit!! The only thing that truly saved my life was that I had an Oakworks massage table in my hatchback.

The fireman came to me and said he wanted to take me to the hospital to get checked out, and that I had to sign off that I wasn't hurt. I proceeded to a massage therapy class. By the time I arrived and sat down on the floor, I realized I was hurt, as my sacrum began pulsating. Later in the evening as I lay in bed, I pressed along the right side of my breast bone to ease the pressure in my chest. I felt the muscles and the thoracic spine move 3/4 of an inch to the right. In shock and probably not sure of what to do, I remembered when I was 12 and what that doctor told me to do to deal with that pain from the heart catheterization, as he extracted the catheters from my groin area, "Hold your breath!" I knew that didn't work! I felt like I was going to die that day!

Now 25 years later, I decided to cry silent tears instead but believe it played havoc on my entire body and mind. All that pain. I was like a good soldier dutifully entering war. It was intense!

Thankfully, I was a massage therapist and had been training and working with injuries. What I was learning was about shifting the way I had cared for my health and wellbeing. It probably saved my life!

One of the classes that inspired me was a Craniosacral Therapy class from now the late, John E. Upledger, DO, OMM (1932-2012). He said during his classes, "The body heals faster using more than one modality at one time." I heard that message loud and clear. After my car accidents, I started implementing the idea of integration toward my healing journey home to myself. It helped me overcome the traumas by re-balancing my body and mind. It helped to calm my nervous system for homeostasis. Each new process was exactly what I needed. I used acupuncture and homeopathy, chiropractic, massage therapy, craniosacral therapy, and energy work.

Then, I saw another therapist who practiced BodyTalk™ System, founded by John Veltheim. After my accident, I had short term memory issues and had to write everything down. BodyTalk™ helped with balancing anxiety, stress, trauma issues, overwhelm, comprehension, following directions, listening better, whiplash issues, and the frustration of not being able to remember; even following simple dance moves were hard to follow. It helps the parasympathetic nervous system to relax after receiving the BodyTalk™ sessions, my pain levels were down between visits. Soon after, I could remember without writing everything down. It took a while for my body to re-establish the communication with the cells of my body. I was vibrating and shaking sporadically for seven years after my car accident, but eventually it got balanced. This time around, I was designing my wellness journey with practitioners either referred or whom I knew personally. The team was at separate locations. Now I truly knew what the late Dr. Upledger meant. As I tried it with my body first, I knew I could begin implementing that type of therapy with my clients, as I knew it worked wonderfully.

I want to provide pain relief for people who have been traumatized in a quick, non-invasive manner. BodyTalk™ is designed to do just that in a tailor-made way. It works on the whole person and provides an opportunity to recover from pain in a gentler manner, and making it an easier journey. I would hope if you were touched by this story, then contact me. Then I have contributed to helping the world heal, one person at a time. Maybe when we are at peace, then world peace will be an acceptable way of being.

Blending massage therapy and BodyTalk™ therapies together really is an excellent way to heal by bringing balance to the whole body. But there may be other treatments that are needed. Learning about your fellow practitioner's skills and services offered will open more doors for you and your client. Research and use their therapies personally. Then you will know exactly how they work and how beneficial someone else's treatments will be for your future clients.

It was a blessing that I moved to Florida and followed my true heart's calling, which lead me to walk down a path less traveled! Thankfully, I listened inside to that wee voice and never stopped, as it has saved my life.

I would also welcome helping children who want to increase their self-expressive abilities. I believe I can help in this manner. When we have head trauma, bringing balance back is essential, as this is a neuroplasticity function that works well within this approach. We forget what our gifts to the world really are after trauma, or interaction with our environment. If I can help by bringing creativity back, then people can shine and explore their true, creative nature, fulfilling their heart's desire.

Being a resource to help people get well from pain is one of the reasons I truly love using the BodyTalk™ System approach to health. BodyTalk™ is a non-invasive, holistic modality that focuses on the whole person, and their unique story to reveal the underlying causes for "dis-ease." When the body is under stress, it isn't communicating to other parts of the body as well as it could. The BodyTalk™ practitioner starts building a formula within the body that it wants to be addressed. Once it is formed, we (practitioners) tap on the head, heart, and gut to create balance. Then, the parts may begin to function on the physiological and the psychological aspects of the individual, addressing their unique story to reveal the underlying causes for "dis-ease." It is designed by your body to bring conscious balance within the cells of your body to the different parts of your body. When there is miscommunication, the cells are not communicating; "dis-ease" is present. Then, the ability to self-heal is compromised. It can be used alone or integrated within any healthcare systematic approach.

To overcome trauma, to be able to get out from the other side, to even be vulnerable to write this story for you - it is a leap of faith and I am very appreciative for the opportunity to write this today.

I believe that God doesn't make mistakes. He placed me on the earth to teach people that they can heal from the inside out! It is a journey and my wish for all mankind to overcome against great odds that pain and terror can transform your life by returning you to your calm state of mind, peaceful attitude, and begin a joyful journey back to one's heart. Sometimes the journey away from the heart is really the journey to the heart! I truly believe this. In order to truly appreciate your health, stay well. When you are faced with catastrophic and challenging life experiences, be prepared to do whatever it takes; as when it is easy in life, we would be all doing it. When it is harder, remember to take the road less traveled; to find the courage, patience, and ability to move beyond fear to joyful celebration. Once this state of mind is achieved, transformation of one's soulful journey home to one's self can also be achieved. You can then tap into your playful, joyful, self-expressive, and creative self that truly is alive and well, when we have reached the end of our journey home to yourself.

"A journey of a thousand miles must begin with a single step."- *Lao Tzu*
This is very true with my life and my recovery.

What I am the most passionate about is the BodyTalk™ System's
integrated approach that came into my life. It had a profound and
significant impact upon my life! In 1999, it was a life-changing moment
when I discovered the "scar tissues technique" from the BodyTalk™ class.
I felt 30 years of scar tissue release without any pain. Unbelievable! At that
very moment, I knew this was my therapy.

I truly like the gentleness and the fast results that I received when giving or
receiving this work. BodyTalk™ is good for the whole family, seniors,
caregivers, and children of all ages. It is one of the most universal systems
that one can truly do in person or remotely. I saw how much easier it was
for people to get well and made my job easier. For example, when it
balanced the stuck energy of emotions, social, mental, behavior, and
physical aspects, it also creates balance. It can be a life changing moment!
Scar tissues congestion, releasing without any pain from an energetic
platform, it then provides looser tissues for me to address afterwards with
other manual therapies. Clients appreciated the combo sessions that were
integrated to resolve their pain issues.

My specialties grew over time. BodyTalk™ for the last 15 years has been
one of the best ways to help people get out of pain. One of the other
reasons I loved this work is that it can be done on myself when I am feeling
stressed or not feeling well. It can combat pain and I have implemented it
for about 12 years for self-treatments and eight years long distance.

I want you to know you should never give up on your dream of getting
better. You can have a second chance. I did! From receiving care from
other holistic practitioners to rebuilding my core muscles with Pilates to
other manual therapies, like structural bodywork and BodyTalk™. It all
helps the body and mind function better, restoring health and well-being; a
total program that incorporates the whole self truly can be your ticket to
radical well-being!

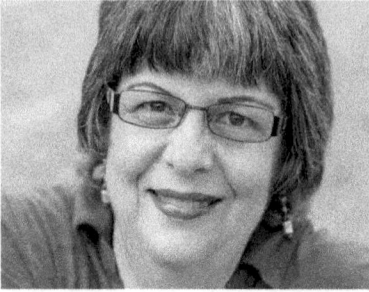

Lisa Seward is a graduate of Suncoast School of Massage Therapy and School of Natural Health, licensed in 1990, certified in 2002 for BodyTalk™ System, and has trained from some of the best in the field of massage therapy. She has studied with the John Veltheim, founder of BodyTalk™, and other top notch teachers. Her practice is a multifaceted, priority-based healthcare approach, which helps bring balance to the whole person. She utilizes other modalities, such as reflexology, shiatsu, direct fascial release, holistic manual lymphatic drainage, TMJ, and chair massage.

Lisa Seward, Licensed Massage Therapist MA10898, Certified BodyTalk™ Practitioner WellnessOptions4U.com
Lisa@WellnessOptions4U.com
www.linkedin.com/in/lisasewardBodyTalk™andmassage

CHAPTER 18

BIRTH OF MY SON LED TO BIRTH OF 100% ORGANIC SKINCARE SEARCH

by Lucie Husarkova, Founder-Hug Your Skin 100% Organic Skincare

My name is Lucie Husarkova and I am originally from the beautiful, historical city Prague, in the Czech Republic. I visited Florida on vacation for many years and fell in love with this state. I love the beaches, the weather, and the friendly people everywhere. My second passion is a holistic approach to living with an aim to buy organic products whenever possible. I have realized that we are each responsible for our own health.

While searching for organic products, I discovered the amazing European skincare company, Inlight. I successfully partnered with Inlight as a distributor in the Czech Republic and Slovakia for three years. Then, I sold my company and created a distributorship in Florida to introduce this luxurious line to the United States and Canada.

But life was not always like this. I had to find my way and make several discoveries on the journey to a healthier life.

Young and unaware of risks of harmful chemicals

Over 20 years ago, I studied at the University of Economics in Prague.

During this time, I had the opportunity to visit Florida and I fell in love with this great country. I decided to someday live here. After my studies, I spent 12 years working for two separate companies in the fast-moving consumer goods (FMCG) industry. I was young and had little interest in cosmetics. I bought mainstream products and didn't pay attention to their ingredients. I had nobody to guide me and explain all the health risks associated with harmful chemical ingredients in beauty products. I did not realize any difference between mainstream beauty products with chemicals and natural or organic products. I lived life like everybody else around me and was focused on my career. The year 2010 approached and I gave birth to my lovely son, Max.

The birth of my son, Max completely changed my lifestyle and priorities

A fantastic, unforgettable day — as any new mum will attest — it also changed my thinking forever. My passion for organic cosmetics and skincare treatments was also born.

Naturally, I wanted the best for my son. So, I sought out ways to give him the best in organic skincare. I studied the ingredients, particularly those products designed for children with sensitive skin. I read about how some are linked to cancer; others disrupt hormones and clog up pores. As a result of my research, I was determined not to use any of these harmful, petroleum-based chemicals on my son's skin! I simply could not imagine putting all those chemical ingredients, connected with such huge health risks, on to the skin of such a little baby. My passion for organic cosmetics had begun.

I couldn't compromise the health of my child

I started to look for a quality product and asked myself two questions:

What is in the product? Is it safe for my child and myself?

My goal? To find 100% organic skincare products.

My search started with pharmacies. The best quality I could find was hypoallergenic products, which literally means products with fewer chemicals. This was not satisfactory for me, so I started to visit specialized health stores. At first, I could only locate items that offered natural or organic ingredients as a percentage of the rest of the product. Naturally, I asked myself the question, *What does the rest contain?* I found out that there is a list of chemical ingredients allowed for use in natural or organic beauty products.

I was unable to find any products that satisfied my requirements in the Czech Republic. I started to travel around Europe, visiting many large organic fairs. One of the big natural expos I visited was in Germany.

I found only one brand offering certified 100% organic skincare

I entered the big hall with hundreds of booths offering natural beauty products. I walked all the way to the corner and the first booth I stopped by was a small booth at the very last row. I came across a small stand where Inlight had a display. I saw they advertised themselves as 100% organic and was intrigued. They informed me they were the only company producing 100% organic products at the fair. Spending the day walking through that massive fair confirmed this. I found nothing else similar to these products. They gave me a test sample of foot and leg balm as I suffered from cracked heels. The results were amazing! After years of searching for a solution, *my cracked heels healed after just 4 days!* The results stunned me and our wonderful partnership began. I finally found what I was looking for!

I started to purchase Inlight skincare from Great Britain for my son, for myself, and for our family members. Later, more and more friends started to use this organic skincare, even those who did not believe that organic skincare can improve their skin condition, and thought only chemicals in skincare can deliver results. Later, in collaboration with two friends, I brought this stunning product into the Czech Republic and Slovakia. We set up a company that offered Inlight organic products and we were able to capitalize on the demand for such high-quality, natural skincare items. Over the next three years, we also became distributors of a couple of other amazing organic brands for make-up, sunscreens, and deodorants from all over the world. We also succeeded in placing those top-quality organic products into pharmacies, specialized beauty shops, and luxury boutiques. Now, many celebrities, including actresses and Miss Czech Republic realized that using skincare and make-up with chemicals on a daily basis does not support healthy skin. They started to use organic products distributed by us.

After three years, I decided to sell my stake in the company. I had bigger ideas. I was ready to introduce this amazing Inlight to the United States, giving American people a chance to experience the benefits of this amazing holistic European skincare brand.

Come with me into a fairytale where skincare smells like an herb garden

I started a new journey. I was introduced to a world of nature that I had not expected. I discovered the secret power of aromatic herbs and oils. After working in logistics for international FMCG companies, this was a radical shift in perspective for me. What took me completely by surprise was how powerful natural products can be when it comes to beauty care. I made a decision and went with my business partner to Cornwall. This is a wild, unspoiled country on the rugged southwestern tip of England where Inlight handcrafts their beautiful and honest products. Doctor Spiezia showed us around his amazing production facilities. This was a miraculous time full of "aha" moments for me. I felt like I was in some kind of fairy tale; one that I want you to visit with me.

Upon our arrival, we received a warm welcome and enjoyed a vegetarian lunch in a blossoming garden. After the meal, Doctor Spiezia invited us into his kingdom - his meticulously clean lab. For years, he has combined herbal wisdom and science to formulate Inlight's 100% organic skincare products. As soon as we walked into the lab, we noticed bags filled with fragrant dried herbs, fruits, and seeds. We stuck our noses in some and inhaled the scents of roses, purple lavender, and orange marigold. We smelled blue cornflower, real vanilla, cocoa, and many other wonderful flowers and herbs. We were surrounded by golden, cold-pressed oils, and I still remember the delicious smell of the coconut oil, jojoba, and evening primrose, as well as the fragrance of the carrot, argan, and macadamia nut. There were many other natural oils too. We enjoyed every second of our visit.

The magic behind the 100% organic skincare of Inlight

Doctor Spiezia showed us a big, round jar filled with a unique mixture of herbs, fruits, and seeds. They were being macerated in a specific mix of cold pressed oils. It was all prepared according to his unique skincare formula, Bio-Lipophilic Matrix. On warmed stones in a glass niche, the herbs suck in the power of the sun and moon for weeks. Some are softened in an oil bath for one lunar month and others for two lunar months. In this way, all the herbs, fruits, and seeds gradually release their powerful healing effects naturally.

Through pressing, we get the final extract. These extracts consist of highly-concentrated oils loaded with nutrients, vitamins, and antioxidants. The gentle pressing process helps them preserve their natural form and efficacy. In this way, we get the bio-active ingredients that are the basis of each natural beauty care product made by Inlight, Dr. Spiezia explained.

Why I became so passionate about healthy cosmetic products

During the past seven years, I've spent a lot of time self-educating about beauty products. I read books by health professionals, visited beauty expos, and talked to beauty professionals. I followed chemical tests executed by various health magazines for cosmetic products. I also started a professional cooperation with several scientists. In one of the publications, the famous Czech scientist, Prof. RNDr.Anna Strunecka, DrSc speaks about the danger from chemical cocktail in the human body and gives us the following examples:

- If you expose 100 rats to a small amount of aluminum, one rat will die.
- If you expose 100 rats to a small amount of quicksilver, one rat will die.
- If you expose 100 rats to a small amount of both toxic ingredients, all 100 rats will die.

An average woman applies 12-16 different beauty products to her skin daily. Each beauty product contains a small amount of chemical ingredients, as allowed by law. But what happens when we expose our body to 12-16 beauty products containing these combined allowed chemical ingredients DAILY? Nobody has ever tested this combination of so many chemicals and nobody can tell us what this mix is doing to our bodies. Why should we risk our most valuable asset – our health?

I have started my own cosmetic research about heavy metals in mainstream skincare with the cooperation of specialized laboratories that utilize huge microscopy. All of my results, including pictures of heavy metals in cosmetics and our bloodstream, are summarized in a clear form in my report, which is available for FREE download from our website: www.hugyourskin.com.

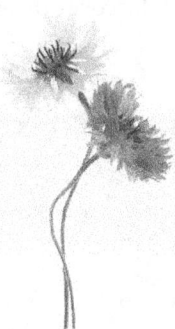

'Only NATURE respects the nature of YOUR skin'

Dr M Spiezia

Why do I believe so much in Inlight?

Before I entered the US market, I performed my own market research. I found many skincare companies offering natural products but I found only two companies that claim most of their products contain 100% organic ingredients. Most of them use water in their formulation. Water is a cheap ingredient and increases the volume of the product. But the presence of water also means the presence of CHEMICAL preservation. This is something that Inlight eliminates.

Doctor Spiezia, skin expert and Inlight formulator, does not compromise on quality. All his ingredients are certified 100% organic and every Inlight product is certified 100% organic. All products are *cruelty free.* The formulations are water-free because water dilutes the powerful formulas, which Dr. Spiezia rejects. Inlight sets a new industry standard – 100% organic.

Dr. Spiezia is an herbalist and homeopathic doctor. His deep knowledge is demonstrated in the right combination of ingredients, which makes the formulations more powerful than the benefits our skin would get from single-ingredient products. He knows exactly which ingredients to combine to achieve the desired result. Inlight is *homeopathic-friendly skincare* and supports a homeopathic healing process.

Enhancing the effect of the products, Inlight beauty combines ancient alchemy and modern science techniques to *maximize the energy and beauty of each ingredient, bringing beauty to life.*

They use eco-friendly packaging to keep the whole process eco-friendly, helping to preserve our planet.

As Dr. Spiezia says, only NATURE respects the NATURE of the skin. There is great truth hidden in these words! It took me almost 30 years to discover that! Join me at www.hugyourskin.com to discover this truth for yourself.

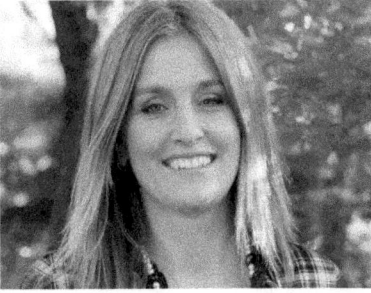

Lucie began her venture into the world of 100% organic skin care upon the birth of her son seven years ago. She founded La Biorganica, distributing organic skin care products in Prague. She also began educating others about the harmful chemicals in beauty products at health festivals and natural expos. In 2016, Lucie moved with her family to Florida and founded Hug Your Skin, bringing the incredible Inlight line with clinically-proven results to the US and Canada. She also conducted her own research about the presence of harmful chemicals in beauty products and our bloodstream. You can find Lucie at www.hugyourskin.com.

HOLISTIC APPROACH

CHAPTER 19

HOLISTIC, INTEGRATIVE HEALING AND COUNSELING
by Michael Whalen MA, LMHC

A Licensed Mental Health Counselor (LMHC) is taught to take to a whole-being orientation, including mind-body-heart-spirit, familial, cultural, and sociological factors, in assessment and treatment of the person in need of assistance. This allows us to join with a person in empathy, understanding, and acceptance of who they are in their circumstance to create a healing milieu.

When I entered graduate school for counseling studies in my early forties, I came with my own set of complementary and holistic experiences that were the result of my own healing journey, begun in my 20's, when I had to face how alcohol was affecting my life. Stopping the use of alcohol and other drugs, 12-step groups, personal counseling to heal childhood familial issues, a move to a vegetarian diet, exercise through running, learning T'ai Chi, yoga, and meditation became foundational practices. I gradually began to heal my body, mind, heart, and spirit.

My thirst for knowledge and growth led to exposure to transpersonal psychology, Adult Children of Alcoholics work, shamanistic healing methods, and indigenous ceremonies, like Sweat-Lodge. I was fortunate to be a part of Harvard's Dr. Herbert Benson's integrative healing initiative using energy fields and chakra balancing. The mythopoetic men's movement helped honor the sacred masculine as a modern man in a changing world. Today, mindfulness meditation is a primary practice which, after more than 20 years, I continue to cultivate and benefit from daily.

I have been fortunate to integrate my schooling in traditional personality theories and counseling methods with a well-grounded holistic foundation in a way that I find both unique and synergistic.

A person can be trained as nutritionist, herbalist, energy healer, counselor or coach, chiropractor, physician, massage therapist, physical therapist, but not practice holistically. The thread that must run through the holistic approach is not only an awareness and inclusion of mind, body, heart/soul and spirit, but also relationship to Earth, its health, and issues of social justice. It is ineffective to address a person's problems while ignoring systemic issues like poverty, racism, sexism, gender bias, environmental climate change, cultural upheaval - all systems in which we live and attempt to thrive.

Inclusive and Integrative, Not Exclusive or Alternative

Healing, from the root to make whole, is different from curing. Healing restores to wholeness and harmony, whereas curing is about eradication of a particular problem or symptom. When we seek to facilitate a person's healing, we assist them to move toward wholeness; to live life optimally.

Western allopathic medicine does not usually incorporate a systems approach to healing. It has separated and siloed areas of functioning into specialties where no one part or practitioner touches another. It has done the same with information and valuable knowledge that exists in other cultures. This has created a very specialized and effective modality for curing symptoms, but not necessarily for optimizing health.

As we approach facilitation of holistic healing, not only are we aware of the mind, body, heart, spirit, and environmental conditions, we must also avoid the mistake of separation and duality in our assessment and approach. We seek unifying, complementary and integrative methods and collaborations using appropriate levels of testing, structural and pharmaceutical interventions, consultations in right circumstance, timing and duration.

Focus on process rather than outcome is much more present oriented in finding fulfillment of any type. To the degree that we can accept conditions as they exist right now as being equal part of the joy of living, whether we perceive it as good or as bad, is the degree to which we can find contentment.

I prefer the terms, "complementary" and "integrative," rather than "alternative" medicine, which creates a 'less than' status. Alternative to what? To the mainstream or "accepted" treatments. Instead, complementary is a term which grants equal side-by-side relationship with the possibility for partnership. "Integrative" creates a synergistic positive impact on the person seeking assistance.

Health Begins in the Mind

Let's look at a story of a person who has had access to an integrative process of professional counseling, complementary and allopathic medicine, and mindfulness to overcome tremendous challenges of circumstance and situation.

Because of confidentiality issues, this is a composite story, not a direct recounting of any one person. All references to actual people are coincidental.

Nervous and Shaky

William came into the office looking pale and shaky, though with a sense of mild bravado that bordered on arrogance. He had a chip on his shoulder that took the form of his kind of sticking his chin out. It was that sense of misplaced bravado that was a telling sign of the outcome of his counseling sessions.

I saw the natural anxiety, shame, and uncertainty that accompanied him as he walked through the door and sat down. I greeted him warmly, acknowledged his discomfort, and complimented his bravery in beginning counseling. As we began to talk, I listened to William with my head, heart, and gut. I heard the story of his latest DUI (I would find out later it was his second in 10 years). But I also heard and saw something more than the assessment form that he had completed could ever reveal.

His written report told about a successful, mid-level professional consultant. It revealed difficulties with siblings and cousins regarding caregiving issues for his father. He was a single gay man.

His main concern was that he knew that it was time for him to stop drinking. He said that this arrest had woken him up. He was not resentful, as some in that situation initially can be, rather, he was determined and had a vulnerability beneath his brave front. As I would find out more and more, William was remarkable, because that fear was accompanied by a fierce determination to be the best he could be. He had just been going about it the wrong way with good reason.

A Reactive Mind

The next session, William began to describe his resentment when people didn't listen to his advice, even though he truly was an expert in his field. But it didn't end at the workplace. The resentment and accompanying aura or arrogance included his family members for their perceived ingratitude for everything that he did for them. He was incensed that he did not get the respect at work, nor the thanks from his family and friends for whom he did so much, that he thought he so much deserved.

As I listened very carefully to William's story, I let him know that I heard, accepted, and empathized with the pain of his expectations not being met. We talked about how he was allowing his happiness to depend on things, people, and circumstances outside of himself. I asked him to consider setting boundaries when it didn't feel right to do things for others.

He also agreed to get a check-up, including blood work to assess liver functioning, as well as levels of Vitamin D, known to facilitate healthy brain functioning and assist with depression. A nutritional consultation was also suggested.

To help reduce stress and build resilience and tolerance for difficult emotions, I taught William mindfulness practices. We discussed how his thoughts were just one part of his experience and to become more somatically aware of the present moment. He could see patterns of his thinking that were leading to anxiety and depression. I knew, through scientifically backed research, that this would begin to tame his reactive brain, making long-term changes in the areas of the brain associated with emotional reactivity and regulation. He would eventually have more success dealing with challenging situations at work and with his family, because he would be less reactive whenever he felt he was being slighted.

William gained insight into how he was not always helping others out of pure generosity, but that he had an agenda as well. He was also doing it for himself in order to get recognition from others to try to fill a very big hole - a lack of self-worth - within. He accepted that he had to take responsibility for getting this need met.

We talked about assertive, blameless, but truthful language and communication with himself, and with those around him. He took on the idea of putting affirmations on his mirror to change his inner beliefs.

"I Finally Feel Safe"

The next session was crucial. William was learning that this was a safe place for him. Again, he came in and spoke about his frustration and resentments. He was angry. Then I asked, "When was the first time you felt this way?" And it happened. William began to describe his 8-year-old self. The little William who was made to feel like he didn't exist by his older brother.

A memory arose of when another boy, a friend of his brother, shoved William from behind. He went down hard. Hitting the hard sidewalk knocked the air out of him. Stunned, he gasped, unable to breath. This was a moment of trauma for that little boy. He struggled for breath. He looked for his older brother for help.

When he turned to look up he saw his big brother laughing, along with the older kid who had knocked him down. This was a moment underlying William's fear and feeling of unworthiness. There were others, but this was a big one. Yes, there were also stories of his overcoming challenges and strengths that were acknowledged as character resources, which was important to his healing as well, but this was a story forged in his mind, body, heart, and spirit that was having lasting impact.

Through mindful, caring therapy William processed through feelings of shame, embarrassment, and the deep pain of betrayal he felt as that little boy. We did an exercise where he, the adult, assured the wounded part of him that the adult William would protect him; would always be there for him.

We also used a leading edge eye-movement therapy, Accelerated Resolution Therapy (ART), to desensitize reactions and restructure the incident in his mind. This quickly helped William's mind to re-envision his story, allowing him to see it differently and lose the troublesome reactions that were triggered whenever he felt he needed to prove himself or when he felt under-appreciated.

That was a critical healing moment in William's healing, freeing him from the reactivity of the trauma to go beyond it. He reported that while he remembered the incident, it seemed distant and had none of the previous emotional charge. He was relaxed and smiling.

William came to understand that his drinking was frequently self-medicating to relieve the feelings of being disempowered. He was taking so many things personally because underneath, he was so tender and was trying to protect himself. He was doing the best he could from the time he was eight. Those weren't all healthy adaptations, but, of course, they were formed by a boy who didn't know other ways of handling the problem. Now that he could see it, he could let his adult self-learn and use the skills necessary to handle it better.

Holistic and Integrative

This was not the only incident or issue that William and I worked on together. We went on to have several more sessions. He also continued his attendance at AA, which he said was very helpful for him. But from that session onward, William began to make changes that were holistically related to his self-care. He improved his diet and nutrition. We explored his sleep patterns and the effect of his unusual work hours on him, physically and socially. He adjusted his schedule. He was more careful to keep in touch with friends through lunches or other outings and planned more carefully. He began to exercise again. He took up the notion of doing things to care for himself and to listen to the "little William" within. He reported he could see that he was looking better and feeling better.

William took important steps toward repairing relationships with those around him. Because he wasn't trying to get a sense of self-worth outside of himself by doing things for others, he began to say "no" and to ask other members of his family to step up in the care of his father. He had some direct and difficult conversations with his partner, as well as his sister and his father.

He spoke with them from a position of equal footing. He made amends for his arrogance and poor behaviors of the past. He talked with them about the way he felt, letting them know that he had a need to feel respected and made specific requests for changes they could consider.

He had learned how to respect himself, to join with his heart, and to live again with spirit. He described an "awakening" in which he seemed to be seeing things in color again. He continued to go to 12-step meetings and stayed committed to being clean and sober, eating well, taking care of his body and surroundings, setting boundaries, and asking directly for what he needed. He returned to church to sing in the choir. Eventually, he also chose to go back to school to further his career goals. He did these things not because he had to, but because he realized this was how he could keep his promise to keep the child-within safe and to live optimally.

This remarkable result may not happen with everyone, nor always so quickly. William's recovery is the product of being able to listen deeply and compassionately, acknowledging him as he was; to point out, without judgment, the damage he was doing to his body and relationships by drinking so heavily and the likely result were he to continue. William learned that he could hold his vulnerability with tenderness and appreciation. He learned to take responsibility and hold himself accountable. William's bravery, tenacity, and commitment to restoring his whole being in mind, body, heart, and spirit were the main features in his regaining his health and himself.

This result is holistic and integrative. Medications were not required, though anti-depressants may have been considered if the healing had not occurred so fluidly, or if the depression was persistent.

As leading edge research develops, experienced counselors employ ever more integrative practices. Neuroscience research has shown that mindfulness can change the brain, grow gray matter, and counter aging-related decline; and that well-being is a trainable skill. Mind-body research into digestive biomes and the brain reveal links between nutrition, gut microbes, and neurotransmitters influencing depression and well-being. Trauma research explores the role of vagus nerve toning in resilience. Eye movement therapies like ART provide rapid resolution for military and other PTSD/trauma survivors. Heart resonance biofeedback can help people with chronic anxiety.

These new discoveries, and more, are available to experienced licensed mental health counselors for the benefit of our clients. It is an honor and privilege to be part of any person's healing journey. It is with deep gratitude that I share with others the holistic, integrative healing I received through many caring hands and hearts.

Unfortunately, there are many more like William. A National Center for Mental Health Promotion and Youth Violence Prevention survey showed that 60% of adults report experiencing abuse or other difficult family circumstances during childhood, and 26% of U.S. children will experience a traumatic event before they turn four. Four in every 10 U.S. children say they have experienced physical assault in the past year. (www.promoteprevent.org/content/childhood-trauma-and-its-effect-healthy-development) It is with deep respect for all the processes of integrated healing that I wish every person best wishes on their daily quest for well-being.

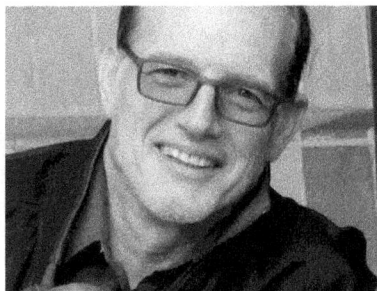

Michael is dedicated to being with others on the daily quest to live life optimally in a healthy relationship with self, family, community, planet, and Spirit. His services help relieve anxiety, move past depression, go beyond trauma, optimize your life and work. He is a 20+ year mindfulness practitioner teaching MBSR-Mindful Awareness Training courses for focus, calm, clarity, compassion. Michael is also an engaging speaker and trainer for conferences, business, and organizations: Time Magazine Customer Services, Johns Hopkins Children's Hospital, Pinellas County School System, Florida Mental Health Counselors Conference, and Florida National Social Workers Association. Host of DayQuest Life! Radio Hour - stories of people who listen for and answer Life's Call.

Michael Whalen M.A., LMHC
www.DayQuestLife.com
Michael@dayquestlife.com
727-341-9397

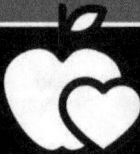

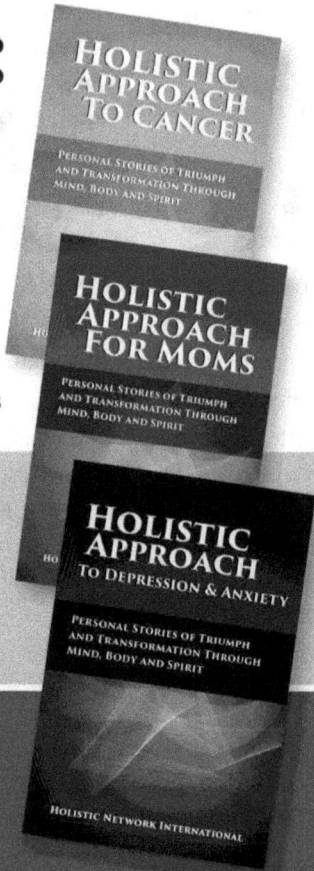

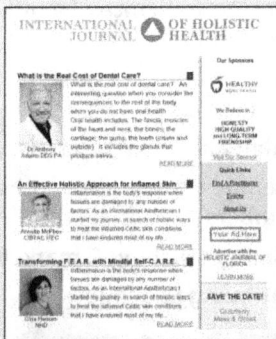

INCREASE YOUR KNOWLEDGE.
ADVANCE YOUR PRACTICE.
BUILD YOUR CLIENTELE.

JOIN HOLISTIC NETWORK INTERNATIONAL

BENEFITS OF MEMBERSHIP

- Collective influence of multiple modalities
- Complementary business partnerships
- Patient and client referrals
- Leverage experience of other members
- Business coaching & marketing
- Continuing Education

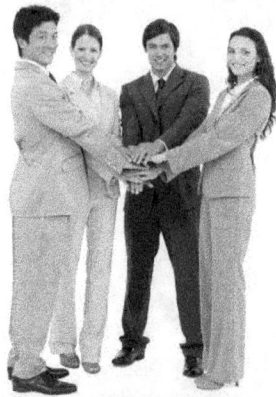

VISIT US ONLINE: HOLISTICNETWORKINTERNATIONAL.COM

"I am a dentist who is looking for alliances to serve others. It is my goal, hope and aspiration that cohesive groups can be organized. The very best way to accomplish this is awareness of each other and formation of alliances. I know of no better tool or group than Holistic Network International. This group is on a mission to serve countless human beings through the organization of others. It doesn't get any better than that." - Anthony J. Adams, DDS, PA

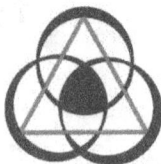

HOLISTIC NETWORK INTERNATIONAL

www.ingramcontent.com/pod-product-compliance
Lightning Source LLC
Chambersburg PA
CBHW052213270326
41931CB00011B/2334